Praise for *Emptying the Nest*

"In *Emptying the Nest: Getting Better at Goodbyes*, Morgan Baker weaves together big emotions and life's minutiae in a way that reminds us that a full life is in the details. *Emptying the Nest* speaks openly of loss and depression while also celebrating the importance of love, family, and self-care to move past the hard times. It is a heartfelt testament to the value of being compassionate with oneself, even in one's darkest moments."

–Myriam Steinberg, author of award-winning graphic memoir *Catalogue Baby: A Memoir of (In)fertility*

"When the reliable world wobbles and spins off its axis, when change upends our lives, the journey to grasping our new reality and one's own new purpose in it is painful, confusing, and long. In *Emptying the Nest*, Morgan Baker has gone into that confusion and pain and left us a trail from bewilderment and sadness to clarity and renewal, from dissolution to resolution. This book is balm and encouragement for all who are unsettled by their losses, stunned by how much they hurt, surprised by intractable sorrow."

–Richard Hoffman, author of *Love & Fury*

"Not only is this inspiring and courageous memoir filled with love, but its sentences are also infused with wisdom, warmth and wit. What began as a fun family thing to do—breeding her beloved dog, Spray—turns into a road to self-discovery for Morgan Baker."

–Delia Cabe, author of *Storied Bars of New York*; Senior Affiliated Faculty of Writing, Literature & Publishing at Emerson College

"How do we frame the story of our lives, measuring the past and finding our way forward just as our worst fears seem to be on the horizon—especially the departures of those we love most? In this forthright, courageous, reflective, and funny memoir, Morgan Baker shows the way. No sugarcoating or glossing for the lessons of love, sadness, joy, and change that are the real deal and appear from some surprising corners, like the litter of ten puppies born at her home. Who can't learn something from a seemingly dead newborn who comes to life in your husband's hands? A tender, beautifully written, and life-affirming guide!"

–Vicki Constantine Croke, author of *Elephant Company: The Inspiring Story of an Unlikely Hero and the Animals Who Helped Him Save Lives in World War II*

"As Morgan moves through transitions that necessitate goodbyes, creates quilts to mark those transitions, and navigates the depression that strikes her as her dog and human families change shape, I relived my own family's transitional years in a deeply emotional way. Morgan's narrative moves back and forth through time, each of her memories a thread connecting to the next, each so filled with heart and often sadness."

–Betsy Leahy Morton

"Morgan Baker's sparkling debut, *Emptying the Nest: Getting Better at Goodbyes*, is a candid, woven-with-love account of mothers, daughters, family, and quilting. Morgan effortlessly weaves themes of love, loss, and separation between mothers and daughters as her girls work to fly the nest, and she works to survive it. Both heartwarming and wry, Morgan's prose is authentic and resonant, her story a field guide to next chapters in life."

–Jacquelin Winter, writer and Pushcart nominee

"As a mother of one daughter (who is also getting ready to start college and who also suffers from anxiety and depression), this memoir is both beautiful and deeply touching. Also, as a veterinarian and fur-mom to six cats and one golden retriever, this is the absolute embodiment of what I adore about Morgan and about dog-people! Morgan's writing is so personal and poignant. This book fills one with the joy of human and fur motherhood, and with the beauty and heartbreak that can be present in loss and change. It is so full of love and hope! I absolutely devoured this book and was very deeply touched by its pages!"

–Dawn Binder, VMD, mother and veterinarian

"I can't remember the last time I read a memoir so quickly. Morgan Baker's *Emptying the Nest: Getting Better at Goodbyes* was a page-turner you couldn't pry out of my hands until the very last word. Baker candidly addresses her battles with depression as she takes the reader on the raw emotional journey of sending her daughter to school and parting with a litter of puppies her dog birthed at home. As the mother of a college freshman and a dog lover, I was captivated by the author's journey. I love how she weaves the experiences of her daughter and the puppies into a rich account of her internal struggle to say goodbye and handle change."

–Jennifer Lovy, blogger and freelance writer

"Morgan Baker's *Emptying the Nest: Getting Better at Goodbyes* is an honest and captivating story of a family—the challenges, triumphs, and losses that occur; and the redemptive power of love, of both humans and dogs, that provides the necessary foundation for reimagining our futures when confronted with inevitable change."

–Deborah Conrad

To

Matt, Maggie, Ellie, and Jay
for showing me love is bigger than a pie

and

Splash, Spray, Ezzie, Mayzie, and Lily
for your unbridled joy

CHAPTER ONE

I suck at goodbyes, separations, and transitions. Sometimes, I sneak to bed to avoid saying goodnight to my family. When our oldest daughter, Maggie, headed off to college—a big transition—I expected to struggle. And struggle, I did.

Maggie and I stood by Matt's blue station wagon in the parking lot in front of her new college dorm. The trunk and roof rack were empty. We had finished unloading boxes and bags of clothes and bedding for Maggie's freshman year. Maggie, Matt, Ellie, and I sweated in the August sun.

An accomplished field hockey goalie, Maggie arrived at the empty campus two weeks before the crush of students and parents. I hugged her, trying to be brave. "I love you."

Maggie pushed me away into Matt. "Take her," she said. "I can hear the warble in her voice." Her long, dark ponytail swayed as Maggie walked away to stand alone on the steps, dressed in jean shorts and a tank-top for the steamy August day.

I had practiced saying goodbye with our litter of puppies earlier in the year, but seeing nine puppies move on to forever homes was very different than saying goodbye to Maggie. I'd prefer to say I didn't get depressed after she stood at the top of her dorm's stairs, looked over her shoulder and waved goodbye, that then I took some meds, did some therapy, and presto, everything was great. I wish that had been the case.

But that isn't what happened.

Separation is tough work, and I'd never been good at it. It didn't matter if I was leaving Matt to hang out with former college roommates for a weekend or if one of my daughters was going to camp for a few weeks. Watching them pack shorts and sunscreen and load their duffle bags in our station wagon for the drive to their respective camps made me sad. I missed them and didn't know what to do without them. But, I was excited for them as we unpacked their duffle bags, put those same shorts away, and toured the site to see where they'd be doing arts and crafts. Driving away and watching them wave goodbye, I wondered if I'd done the right thing, encouraging this thing called independence.

I stressed, stewed, worried, and wondered if everyone, including me, was going to be okay. Regardless of whether my kids left or I went away for a friends' weekend, I wondered if they would thrive in their solo experiences and if I could enjoy my time without worrying about them. Would we all reunite as a family unit, tighter than before?

Perhaps my distaste for parting stemmed from the day in 1968 when my father walked my mother, brother, baby sister, and me onto a Pan Am flight from New York to London. He handed my brother and me a Steiff lion and lioness—each with a £20 note strapped to its belly. Clutching my stuffed lioness, I felt the weight of my father's love in my lap, cozy and comforting. That warm feeling chilled as he walked away down the plane's center aisle.

At nine years old, I experienced the end of our family as I knew it.

I was a New Yorker, until that flight when I wasn't, although I would return to the city for weekends with my father, and to see friends when I was much older.

That separation surfaced as a big surprise. One day after Christmas when I was in fourth grade, my mother and father had sat my seven-year-old brother and me down at the round dining room table, and Daddy said, "Your mother is going to move with you and your baby sister to London. You will go to school there, and I will come visit."

That's all I remember.

When I visited London after college with my college roommate years later, I was struck by what my mother had done. What had possessed her? Why so dramatic a move? She had been in her mid-thirties with three kids.

I never got the chance to ask her, but divorce in the 1960s was a shameful event. She was probably mortified, and London seemed reasonable because my grandmother had friends in London on whom my mother could rely, and it was far enough away that my parents couldn't see each other even if they wanted.

My brother and I finished off our second and fourth grades at the American school there. My mother hired a sitter to help care for the baby during the day, and my brother and me after school.

My father visited us once during a business trip. He had traveled to different countries, including Russia, and he gave me a gold bear charm from there to add to my charm bracelet.

When we returned from London eight months later, we didn't go home to New York. We went directly to my grandmother's on Martha's Vineyard. There, we played roof ball (chucking a tennis ball onto the roof and then running to catch it as it tumbled back to the ground) and tennis. We ate wildly rich food made by my grand-mother's housekeeper, who cooked with cream and butter. Sitting on Grandma's back porch, we watched the ever-changing sunset of orange and red over the field and Vineyard Sound.

Grandma's house would remain my safe haven for years to come. It was the one constant in my life.

For the rest of my life, I dreaded separation, clinging tightly to friends and family. When I went off to Vassar—almost four hours away—I lasted one semester before returning home to my mother and stepfather's house, where they had just welcomed their new baby, Will. I was convinced he was my replacement. After all, his arrival did coincide with my departure.

I spent much of that first semester self-medicating, as they say. I thought I was having fun, meeting new people and hanging out in the campus bar, but I was really hiding from myself and others how lonely and scared I was.

I hadn't been happy or particularly friendly in our reconfigured family. I was mad at my parents and took it out on my stepfather. It wasn't his fault my parents were divorced or that I missed my father.

My memories of that time flit like fireflies. He and I got into a lot of fights, most of which I have blocked out. I was rude to him and didn't appreciate any of the sacrifices he had made, specifically mar-rying a woman with three children. We didn't always see eye to eye on issues, but he stayed with my mother until she died at sixty-nine.

As an adult, I'm embarrassed by my behavior, but as a mother who raised two teenage girls, I have more compassion for the thirteen-year-old who experienced divorce, several moves, and a bunch of parental remarriages.

After Will entered our lives, my brother, sister, and I started calling our stepfather "Dads" rather than John.

Over time, Dads and I became good friends, but more importantly he was my second father. When I married in 1988, I walked down the church aisle alone, my two fathers, both of whom were significant figures in my life, flanking me behind. And in 2005, he and I teamed up to take care of my mother when she was sick.

But in 1976, I believed love was like a pie with only so much to go around—the more people jousting for a piece, the smaller mine would be. With motherhood, I finally understood that love is limitless. Only then did I see how I could just keep loving and loving, that love didn't fit into a jigsaw puzzle with an edge around it. Love is truly boundless, like sunrises and sunsets that spread color across the horizon.

As Maggie prepared to leave the warm and cozy home I had created, I worried about how I would fare. Maggie's last year at home was going to be hard, but I signed up for every volunteer opportunity at her school. I fed the kids pizza once a week and helped throw a Valentine's Day party.

But what really kept us all distracted from how much our family was to change, were our dogs—all twelve of them.

Our first dog, Splash, joined our family when Maggie was seven. She had begged for one, and we put it off as long as we could, telling her she could have one when she turned seven. So, when she asked where it was on her birthday, we quickly researched and decided on Portuguese water dogs (PWD). Matt was allergic to dogs, cats, horses, and an army of foods. PWDs cause fewer allergies in humans than other breeds because they have hair, not fur.

No dog is completely hypoallergenic, but PWDs seemed to be the best choice. Maggie, as it turned out, also became allergic to dogs.

Books, websites, and dog experts warned us how much work PWDs required and suggested they may not be right for first-time dog owners, let alone a family with young children.

Matt and I downplayed some facts: that PWDs like to be with their owners constantly; are highly energetic, mouthy (ours liked to chew tables, eyeglasses, and stuffed animals) and strong-willed (which helped them back when they aided fishermen in Portugal's Algarve area). According to the American Kennel Club (AKC), they herded fish into nets, retrieved broken nets, and acted as aquatic couriers from boat to shore or between boats. We ignored the Portuguese water dog website, which said they were "resistant to fatigue." They are working dogs, and they need and want to stay busy.

We paid attention to the characteristics that appealed to us: they are friendly, cheerful and loyal, and they let children climb on them and pull their hair. They seemed interesting and similar to the dogs that Matt had as a child: a Labrador and a Newfoundland. We figured we could make it work. We trusted each other.

Yes, my family history made separating hard, but something else also factored into my challenges. In fifth grade, Maggie changed. Before, she had been a social girl who loved school. She had many friends with whom she played at school and on weekends. Suddenly, that girl was nowhere to be found. She didn't hang out with her friends, and it looked like they had all ditched her.

I went to the school psychologist to say Maggie wasn't the same kid, and I didn't get it. The psychologist told me not to worry, these things happen. I knew she was wrong. I knew my daughter. And, unfortunately, I was right.

One evening, her fifth-grade teacher called to say they'd had a program that day on how to recognize inappropriate behavior. I didn't like where this was going. Maggie, to her credit, had disclosed about a "kiss" from an older male babysitter. We didn't really know this person. Not that it matters. Matt was at a year-long fellowship at Harvard, and they provided sitters for all the fellows' children through a service they hired. Like most predators, the sitter had encouraged her to keep it secret. Until, one day, Maggie, again to her credit, told him she couldn't keep the secret anymore. He stopped showing up for his regular sitting job. I'm not sure if Maggie pushed her friends away to control her world, or because she didn't want to share what had happened.

In high school, she made new friends, and much later, in her twenties, she did reconnect with many of her elementary school friends. Around the same time, and after a lot of therapy, Maggie said, "Mummy, it happened. I survived, and I'm stronger for it." Those words were a gift.

For years, I worried about her, wanted to protect her, and felt responsible for what had happened. But before her successful climb to strength and survival, she was lonely (especially in middle school). She read books, watched movies, and snuggled with Splash—her best friend. He remained so for years, despite his unattractive habits like barking at trucks and motorcycles, chasing school buses up our street, and occasionally biting a few people. When others thought we should part with him, I stood my ground. He was Maggie's.

I also didn't understand that Splash was lonely, too. Like me, he didn't like separation. I drove the girls to school frequently, and as we turned onto its street, Splash whined, cried, and lay on top of the girls in the back seat. Danny—part of the maintenance crew and carpool checker—laughed every day listening to Splash's painful lament as the girls jumped out of the station wagon. Maggie and Ellie often laughed with Danny, but they also were quick to get on the playground so as not to be embarrassed by their dog.

Before they were jumping out of the car, they were babies, dependent on me. But even after they were born, lying in the hospital with each of them, my life was forever changed, and they would separate bit by bit for the rest of their lives.

I wanted them to learn how to forge forward independently into their own lives, but it meant letting go of them, little by little. My role was to support them and encourage them with little nudges as appropriate, when instinctively all I wanted was to hold them.

Sending them off to preschool and kindergarten would be a precursor to the big send-off, when they went to college and left me for good.

CHAPTER TWO

I make quilts to celebrate transitions in my family and friends' lives.

I made my first quilt thirty-six years ago (in my twenties) as a wedding gift for a college roommate. I didn't know what I was doing, but I wanted to mark this occasion with something personal. I knew how to make pillows, so I had figured making a quilt couldn't be that much different. It was. The seams ripped apart not long after my friend's wedding. She and her husband hung it on their wall for a while because it was too delicate to put on the bed. I haven't asked what happened to it since. But, since then, my skills have improved, and I made quilts for her four children and six grandchildren.

Quilts are my way of saying, "I love you, and here is something to wrap yourself up in and move on in your life." The more I made, the better the quilts became.

To mark this big event in Maggie's life, I planned to make her a going-to-college quilt. I wanted to start it before the fall of her senior year of high school, leaving me plenty of time to get it done—at least a year.

But, at Keepsake Quilting (in Center Harbor, New Hampshire) in early September, I didn't know this project was going to be labor intensive and emotionally draining. My younger daughter, Ellie, came with me to select the fabric. Since my kids were toddlers, they have accompanied me into many quilting stores, mostly at The Cambridge Quilt Shop (which is less than two miles away from our home).

Keepsake was the largest quilting store I knew, with aisles and aisles of fabrics and rows and rows of design books. I knew I'd find the fabric for Maggie's going-to-college quilt. Not only did I want it to remind her of the ocean, but I also wanted her to have a part of me.

Maggie loved swimming. She loved the Atlantic Ocean off Martha's Vineyard. She is a strong swimmer and spent hours leaping over and diving under waves and floating on her back.

I pulled out bolts of ocean-themed fabrics with sailboats and lighthouses, but Ellie said, "Mummy, those are icky. They're for kids. Maggie won't like them."

Matt and I, coincidentally, called our mothers "Mummy." It had nothing to do with living in England. Both our mothers grew up in New Haven, so maybe it was a New Haven thing. But, it was more evidence of why we were such a good team. We shared so many similar experiences: divorced parents in the '60s, remarriages, big families, living in Cambridge, and we both graduated from Vassar.

My siblings all grew out of "Mummy" and called her "Mom," "Ma," or later, after becoming a grandmother, "Gabby." Now, I am "Mummy," and I love it.

I wandered the Keepsake aisles some more and discovered the batik fabrics, specifically the blues and greens. An older couple also walking the aisles asked what I was making. I explained my project and tried not to cry.

"Don't worry," the husband said. "They're like boomerangs. They always come back." I smiled with gratitude. This departure might not be as bad as I was anticipating.

Starting the fall of Maggie's senior year, the quilt pieces in varying shades of blue, green and white hung over the railing that kept family and guests from falling down the stairs on our second floor. I took over the dining room. Fabric swatches, cutting boards and my sewing machine reigned. We ate in the kitchen.

As much as I worked on it, it wasn't ready when Maggie left for college. I didn't give it to Maggie until she came home for spring break during her freshman year. This quilt was taking an absurdly long time to make.

Matt said, "I think if you finish it, you'll feel that is your last tie to Maggie." Smart man. The familiar process of measuring, cutting, and sewing kept me busy so I didn't obsess about Maggie leaving, and once she was gone, working on it did keep her close.

In 1991, and again in 1995, I made quilts to welcome my two babies into the world. Matt and I didn't know what we were having either time, so the quilts consisted of colors that could work for a boy or a girl. One was a star pattern in shades of blue and white; the other was an around-the-world pattern with yellows, blues, and whites.

We had two girls.

Maggie bunched her quilt up and used it as a lovey. By the time she left for college, I had patched it several times, but it was still full of rips and holes. Ellie, on the other hand, slept under hers, smoothing it out so there weren't any wrinkles. Hers faded with time, but it is still in one piece.

Maggie was, and is, a creature of comfort. She likes to bury herself under blankets and enjoys being cozy. Ellie also likes being cozy, but she was, and is, more systematic and ordered. We didn't know this for years, but her tendency for order was an indication of the obsessive-compulsive disorder she was diagnosed with later.

Even their births were indicative of their personalities. Maggie loved being first in line at school, and she was competitive in sports and board games. She came a week early, eager to get into the world. Ellie, on the other hand, is concerned about rules and not breaking them. Her moral compass has always been strong. While I went into labor with her on the day before she was due, she waited until the appropriate time and came just after midnight on her due date.

My quilts have been used as playmats for babies, as lovies in daycare, as sleeping pals and even wall art. When I hear that a three-year-old brings his quilt with him to nursery school, I swell with pride. More than twenty years after I gave a baby quilt to a friend's daughter, she showed me the pieced-together remnants. It wasn't recognizable, but I knew she had loved it for a long time. I usually make a few quilts a year, depending on how many babies are born and who is getting married.

But just as getting ready to say goodbye to Maggie was not part of my normal, the pandemic in 2020 and not seeing Maggie or other family members for more than a year was also not part of normal. I missed them and tried to find meaning in the year of lockdown. Quilting helped. I made fourteen.

Over the years, Matt and my daughters have become more adept at looking at the fabric I bring home and imagining it as a quilt. "That is beautiful," Matt—the leader of my fan club—said as I pieced together a quilt of pastel colors for our nephew and his new wife. Choosing patterns and colors is challenging and fun. For years, I resorted to the same-old patterns I knew well. But as time went on, and especially during lockdown, I pushed myself to experiment with new ones. I always tried to use colors the recipients would like. Blues and whites for a niece and her new husband; turquoise and teal for another niece and husband; and greens, blues, pinks, and reds for babies.

In 2009, during her junior year, before I was even imagining her quilt, Maggie visited many colleges. These visits were fun and distracting. Matt took her on most of them, as my teaching schedule at Emerson conflicted with her spring vacation. She and I took a couple of long weekends. On one, we headed north from Boston to see Skidmore, UVM and McGill.

In Montreal, Maggie sat in on an English class, while I sat in a recliner in the coffee shop of an off-campus bookstore, reading. Then we took a self-directed tour of McGill's dorms (unlike other schools we visited, McGill's guided tour only covered the academic buildings).

Maggie complained as we walked up a long hill on a very cold day. "I don't want to stay for the real tour," she said. She had been surprised by how large the English class was and how little the students discussed the reading material.

The college counselors at her high school had advised parents to keep their opinions to themselves. The tours and college search were the students' experiences. Maggie was supposed to "drive the bus" and come to her own conclusions about each college she visited. It was hard to keep my opinions to myself. I loved to talk and share, but I didn't want to influence Maggie, so I kept my trap shut and simply repeated what she said, much to her aggravation.

"I understand you don't want to stay for the tour," I panted, following her up the icy hill. "Look at how close you'd be to the hospital if you had an allergic reaction." I pointed out the neighboring institution.

Not only was I afraid of how much I would miss Maggie, but I also wasn't ready to relinquish control over her safety. As a baby, Maggie had been diagnosed with life-threatening food allergies, particularly to tree nuts and peanuts. Later, she developed allergies to legumes and sesame as well.

When she was eleven months old and in her high chair, I had slathered peanut butter on some crackers. I was thrilled she liked it. I lived on peanut butter and fluff as a kid and still indulged in those sandwiches. I watched her eat the first cracker. She picked up a second with a big smile. I ran off to the bathroom, and when I returned, she was a different child. Her face was swollen, her eyes were almost shut, and she was covered in hives.

Maggie gulped some liquid Benadryl I gave her, and then I called the pediatrician. The answering service told me the office was at lunch, but not two minutes later, I got a return phone call. "Is she breathing?" That's when I knew this was serious.

I protected Maggie and educated her school, friends, and family about these allergies, initiating changes at school and more awareness in general. But I couldn't protect her at college. It was time to let go.

"I don't like these dorms," Maggie said as we walked from building to building in Montreal.

"I understand you don't like the dorms," I echoed.

"Let's just go," she said as we shivered in the March air. "Don't you agree?"

"I understand you want to go." If it was chilly now, I wondered how cold it would be in the middle of January…

"Mummy. Stop. What do you think?"

I thought she might punch me.

"I think you need to decide what you want to do."

We left and drove to Burlington, Vermont, where we stayed with my youngest brother, Will, and his wife, Stacey. We toured UVM's windy and huge campus. Again, not a great fit for Maggie. Even though she wasn't interested in any of the schools we visited, the visits were useful as she began to discern what she liked and what she didn't.

I relished this time with her, where she was trapped in my car and we listened to her playlists—with Coldplay and the Backstreet Boys—driving through Vermont. I tried to live in the moment and not project into the future, thinking about how empty my car would be in a year.

A few weeks later, Matt took her to New York and Pennsylvania. They watched tour guides walk backwards at nine schools, some of which Maggie eventually applied to. She didn't even get out of the car at other stops, telling her dad to keep going.

While some students fall in love with a particular school and apply early decision, Maggie didn't have that experience. She didn't go gaga over any college. She found something wrong with each one she visited. Her application process dragged on, lasting into May of her senior year, when she had to decide between the schools that had admitted her and whether she would play field hockey at any of them.

CHAPTER THREE

We added our second dog, Spray, when Ellie was thirteen, two years before I took Maggie to college. Ellie also struggled with friends and school. She had an overwhelming case of obsessive-compulsive disorder (OCD) that her third- and fourth-grade classmates didn't understand, but it gave them a great reason to tease her.

Mental health issues in my family and Matt's are like the chocolate chips in a Toll House cookie: plentiful. I had fought with depression several times in my life, and various relatives had experienced significant challenges too, including depression, bipolar disorder, anxiety, and who knew what else lurked under the surface. People don't often wear their diagnoses pinned to their shirts.

When Ellie was eight, she said, as I put her to bed one night, smoothing her quilt over her, "Mummy, you know why I repeat myself all the time?"

"No, why?"

"The monsters make me do it."

And then I knew. Her idiosyncrasies were not just annoying behaviors; something was definitely off. She was fighting something, but she didn't know what it was. Neither did I.

She was officially diagnosed with OCD, but that didn't help her when the kids in her class found her habit of tapping her foot repeatedly confusing and irritating. OCD is often misunderstood, and not only by kids. It is more than a quirky trait about being neat and washing your hands. It is complicated and devious. To say you have OCD without being diagnosed can be offensive to those who understand the severity this illness can wreak on people.

According to the National Institute of Mental Health: "OCD is a common, chronic, long-lasting disorder characterized by uncontrollable, recurring thoughts (obsessions) that can lead people to engage in repetitive behaviors (compulsions)."

Although everyone worries or feels the need to double-check things on occasion, the symptoms associated with OCD are severe and persistent. These symptoms can cause distress and behaviors that interfere with day-to-day activities. People with OCD may feel the urge to check things repeatedly or perform routines for more than an hour each day as a way of achieving temporary relief from anxiety. OCD can never be eradicated from a person's life, but patients can learn how to manage it. If untreated, however, these behaviors can disrupt work, school, and personal relationships and can cause feelings of distress.

Ellie fought OCD, or "the monster," for years. She worried about her family's safety, especially if any of us were driving, and obsessed about Matt and Maggie's life- threatening food allergies.

When she was young, Ellie countered her obsessions with compulsions that manifested as repetitious behaviors, always in even numbers. When she or another family member left the house, she said "I love you" two, four or six times. This, she thought, would keep her family safe. She read slowly because she reread sentences two or four times. She also tapped her feet and hands against table-tops and legs. If her right foot tapped the table leg twice, then the left foot tapped twice. OCD also demanded that Ellie ask for reassurance constantly. This is not uncommon.

Understanding OCD and its tendencies was helpful to the family, but that didn't mean I didn't get frustrated when, as she got ready for bed, she sat in my lap and said, "Am I going to die tonight?" While reassuring would have been so easy, I didn't want to feed the monster. I practiced saying, "I don't know. What do you think?"

So, when Ellie asked for a dog to help with her anxieties, Matt and I agreed. We thought a dog might provide a sympathetic ear for her worries, or at least a nonjudgmental friend to hang around with on weekends. I wanted, and was determined to get, a calm female. I did not need another Splash.

I was more careful with my research. I looked for an experienced breeder, who bred for temperament, not just appearance. After months of perusing websites and making phone calls, I found a couple in Rhode Island who put us on their waiting list for a litter due at the end of July. Right after the puppies were born, however, the breeder called to say two of them had died and they no longer had one for us.

I was crushed. I went back to searching for another litter.

A couple of weeks later, the breeder, Sandy Nightingale, called to say a buyer had backed out. If we were still interested, a female puppy was available. Yes, we were.

Matt, Ellie, and I drove down on a sunny weekend day in late August. Maggie was at a Six Flags amusement park for a birthday party. Ellie was annoyed she had to go for a ride with us. We didn't tell her where we were going. We wanted to surprise her.

"Are you taking me to boarding school?" she asked from the back seat of our station wagon.

"Right, Ellie. Like we would just put you in the car and drop you off at boarding school without discussing it beforehand. No.

We're not taking you to boarding school." I hoped my sarcasm calmed her.

"We're taking you to an audition for a commercial," Matt improvised. Ellie, a budding actor, would have killed for any chance to act anywhere.

"Really?" she asked.

She admitted later that she didn't really buy the audition story either, but it relaxed her enough in the moment.

We drove down a long tree-lined, residential dead-end road in Warren, Rhode Island, and pulled into Jim and Sandy Nightingale's driveway. A mailbox with Portuguese water dogs painted on it stood sentry at the end of their driveway. Ellie missed this detail.

Sandy and Jim came out and introduced themselves, both tall and friendly. We followed them inside to the tiled breezeway in their house, where Ellie saw a playpen on the floor. She looked into it and up at us. "Puppies?" she asked, a huge smile crossing her face. "Puppies?!"

This was worth all the closed doors and hushed conversations with breeders. I had successfully kept the project a secret, and the smile on Ellie's face told me how happy she was just to see puppies, and then to realize one was for her.

Two six-week-old female puppies were available. One was a traditional looking black and white PWD. The other was white with a black eye and rump. Her hair hadn't grown out yet, so she looked more like a white rat than a dog, and I'm not a fan of rats.

Matt and Ellie played with both puppies. The white one licked Matt's toes in his flip-flops and climbed over Ellie's feet. I picked them up and held them, but even though they were both cuddly, I was adamant that we needed the calmer puppy. Sandy assured me the white one was the calmest, even if she did look like a rodent, but

I trusted her judgment. This was Sandy's seventh litter, and she, like most experienced breeders, knew how to read puppy temperaments and how to test them for their traits as well. Dog temperaments—whether passive, stable, confident, aggressive or shy—are a result of both inherited and environmental factors.

Back at home, when we showed Maggie pictures of the puppy, she thought we had lost our minds—I did too. I was not a white dog person. White dogs were for people who knew how to keep their houses and dogs clean. I always thought they were for prissy, frilly ladies—not me.

Photographs of my family (mostly of the girls at various ages) cluttered my house. Framed photos of my daughters in New Hampshire, in Halloween costumes, and at Christmas covered counters, tables, and window ledges. They also hung above door-jambs and on a photo wall down a hallway.

And, much to Matt's dismay, there were elephants everywhere. Elephant candle holders, elephant pillows, an elephant table, elephant bowls and hundreds of miniature elephants made of wood, glass, and silver were also featured on counters, couches, walls, and shelves.

In fifth grade, a boy gave me my first teeny glass elephant, but I really fell in love with elephants when my brother and I went to India when I was fourteen to visit the then-Ambassador's family. My brother was friends with Daniel Patrick Moynihan's son. There, I rode an elephant, saw many, and learned how important family was to elephants.

Since then, I have collected enough elephant items to fill a museum. I have even been gifted several orphaned baby elephants in Kenya. Only now, as a mother, do I understand why elephants are so important to me. They move as family units, and they never leave anyone behind, even sitting vigil with a deceased family member.

To round out our mess, my quilting projects always occupied our dining room. Fabric lay on the table, and half-made quilts hung over the banister from the second floor. We weren't hoarders, but we weren't neat.

Our house is upside down. Our living and dining rooms, along with our kitchen and a small family room, are on the second floor. We live in what was traditionally a Philadelphia style two-family home. For the first six years after Matt and I moved in 1991, we rented out a three-bedroom apartment with one bedroom on the first floor and two on the second. As the kids grew, we incorporated one and then two rooms from the rental into our own unit.

By the time Spray came along, we had absorbed most of the rental, leaving a small one-bedroom apartment that we rented first to the Nieman Foundation, then Matt's aunt lived there when she needed care, and after which a friend's son stayed for four years while he was in graduate school. Jay, Maggie's boyfriend, moved in after that.

I didn't believe we were considering showing or breeding Spray—which was the name we gave the white puppy—so whether Spray conformed to the standards of the breed didn't seem important. The purpose of standards (including gait, temperament, and structure) is to be a guide for breeders and judges. According to the AKC, dogs rarely stand up to every one of them.

We just wanted a family-friendly pet. But apparently, Jim Nightingale and Ellie had talked about showing the puppy. Meanwhile, Matt and Sandy talked about breeding her, and the contract we signed stated we didn't have to spay her. Most contracts are restricted, indicating that the owner will neuter their pup so as to curtail the number of unwanted dogs in the world and to cut down on irresponsible backyard breeders and diseases.

Sandy was right. Not only was Spray the calmest, mellowest, and sweetest dog out there, but also, she was almost human, our person-dog. She was the opposite of Splash. I enjoyed taking Spray for walks around Fresh Pond, the reservoir near our house. I never feared she would attack a runner or chase a bicyclist. "Spray, stay with me," I said. She did. If we neared a puddle or the small pond along the path, and I said to stay or sit, she did—unlike Splash, who dove into an inch of water.

By the time we decided to get Spray, I knew what I was doing. I was getting a friend for Splash and Ellie. A second dog might also give Splash some companionship and make him less lonely. I wondered if perhaps some of his anxiety might have stemmed from being alone so much.

Dogs and humans have complicated and intricate relationships. While dogs rely on humans for physical survival, humans rely on dogs for protection and emotional security. Some people say they get more emotional support from their dogs than their spouses. There have been times when Matt would agree.

Often, that bond is cemented with anthropomorphic projections, because humans treat their pets, especially dogs, like little people. Matt often calls our dogs "his friends," and I often speak for them, changing the intonation and depth of my voice to distinguish who is speaking, me or them. If Matt wants to know if our dogs have been fed, I might say, "Yes, thank you. My kibble was particularly delicious this evening," in a high pitch. Life is more interesting when I pretend to know what's on their minds.

One of Spray's favorite places to lounge was in Matt's chair by the fireplace. There she sat upright like a human, with her front paws draped over the armrest, ready to engage in conversation. She just needed a cigar and a glass of bourbon.

When I came home from teaching at the end of the day, I often found Splash lying in front of Spray's crate in Matt's office, keeping her company and waiting for her to come out and play. Splash, at almost nine, was old enough that he didn't need to be crated anymore. He was house-trained and didn't destroy the house, but Spray was still learning and was apt to chew books, eyeglasses, and chair legs if left alone, so she was crated when we weren't home.

Two dogs weren't much more work than one. In many ways, they were easier to take care of because they entertained each other. I didn't have to worry about getting them all the exercise they needed because they played chase or tug-of-war with toys in the house.

Spray did keep Splash company, but more importantly, she helped Ellie manage her anxiety. Alone in her room, Ellie had a friend to depend on who would listen to her and not judge her for what some of us might have considered irrational thoughts. Ellie fell in love with Spray (or Spray-Spray, as we often called her).

When Spray was six months old, it was time to discuss spaying her. It was also time to plan for Maggie's next phase of life—looking at colleges and figuring out where she might want to go.

Matt thought breeding Spray would be a fun family adventure. I didn't. The idea was irresponsible, and I knew it could lead to some health problems for Spray later. She could develop pyometra (an inflammation in her uterus), or we could potentially find ourselves with dead puppies.

"It'll be fun," Matt said in his office among papers and children's art. "A bonding experience." I stood in the doorway, shaking my head.

What about the cost, the work involved, and the health risks? I asked him over and over.

Along with Spray's risk of breast and uterine cancer, which

would increase the longer we left her intact, I worried about how to incorporate breeding into my life. Spray would be the right age to breed in a year and a half. How could we manage taking care of puppies, Ellie's school and carpool, my job at Emerson College, the twenty-four seven demands of Matt's job and Maggie's college application process?

Breeding is also expensive. Most breeders don't go into breeding to make money. They do it because they love the breed and want to create happy families, and they want to carry the line forward. They're lucky to break even, what with all the cash—several thousand dollars—they need to pay upfront in medical expenses and stud fees, before they see any of it back in sales.

The Portuguese water dog almost died out after they were no longer needed to help fishermen in Portugal. Technology replaced them. By 1930, with almost no PWDs around, a wealthy shipping magnate took interest and started a breeding program. In 1958, two Portuguese water dogs were shipped to the United States, and that started an interest in the breed here. The Portuguese Water Dog Club started in the 1970s, and the AKC recognized the breed in the early 1980s.

PWDs will swim anywhere they can find a body of water, but their working lives were over. They were pets, loyal friends to their owners who swam in lakes, ponds, and the ocean for fun.

If I waited Matt out, he might come to his senses. He'd realize I was right. We didn't know a thing about breeding, and we didn't have the time or money. Matt loved Spray too much to risk her health. Spray was the perfect dog, as he told everyone. We'd hardly had to train her. She knew how to sit and stay intuitively, and she loved Matt back, frequently sitting in his lap.

But, we didn't spay Spray. At least not yet.

CHAPTER FOUR

When Spray turned one the following July, Matt and I still hadn't resolved our disagreement about breeding her. Waiting him out wasn't working.

Our sweet, unflappable vet, Dr. Emara, told me that when Spray went into heat it would probably last for four weeks, with ten active days during which we had to watch her around the clock. She was kicked out of her doggie daycare because we hadn't neutered her, and she couldn't go on walks or to her daily playgroup—when our dog walker, Scott, took Splash and Spray out for several hours with a pack of other dogs. Because she wasn't neutered, it could lead to a problem when male dogs, particularly intact ones, got near her.

Inside, she spotted all over the house—on the white kitchen tiles, the white bathroom tiles, and the sheets and mattress pad on our bed. I did a lot of laundry and wiped up little droplets with rags.

Even more unappealing than the blood, however, was Splash, who took an avid interest in fertile Spray, despite being fixed. I couldn't count how many times he humped her or how many times I yelled, "Off, Splash! Get off, you gross dog."

Most animals only have sex to reproduce. Humans have sex to reproduce and for pleasure, so it's not surprising that we often read into animal behavior much that isn't there, anthropomorphizing their actions. If we did have puppies, how would Spray handle parting with them? Would that kill her, the way I anticipated Maggie's departure for college would affect me?

Part of Spray's cycle also coincided with my annual vacation on Martha's Vineyard. My family has been visiting the Vineyard every summer since my great-great-grandparents stumbled upon it in the 1860s, when—according to family legend—my great-great-grandfather stopped there on a hospital boat after the Civil War.

For most of my childhood, I spent summers with my grandmother in Lambert's Cove, which is a short drive from Vineyard Haven into West Tisbury. In the 1930s, she and my grandfather bought a shingled house trimmed in Nantucket Blue "for a song." They had a picture-perfect view of the Vineyard Sound and Naushon Island from their back porch, and it was a five-minute walk across a meadow and over dunes to the beach.

My grandmother's house provided everything I needed for the summer. She had a clay tennis court with a too-small backstop and too-narrow side alleys where I learned how to make a wicked cross-court shot that was often hard to return. She also had the path to Lambert's Cove beach, where I could be found every day, especially as a teen, swimming or lying in the sun.

Grandma taught me to always carry a book, bathing suit, and a sweater—you never knew when you'd have to wait for a ride or when you'd be invited to the beach or the weather would change.

When my parents divorced, the Vineyard became my grounding spot, and it was where I reconnected with Matt, an old college friend, one summer after I finished getting my master's in professional writing at Emerson College.

I was teaching at Emerson and temping in Boston when he and Bob—another Vassar friend—and Bob's girlfriend, Debbie, took a week's vacation on the island. Bob suggested I hang out with them.

I'm not sure if he had planned on putting Matt and me together, but we fell in love walking on sandy Philbin Beach, dotted with large rocks in the water, up-island in Aquinnah at the easterly tip of the Vineyard. We listened to Earth, Wind & Fire, had dinner with my family, had dinner at Matt and Bob's rental, and discussed the overuse of the word "that" on a beach across the road from the Abel's Hill Cemetery in Chilmark. Years later, my mother was buried there. We played Wiffle ball in the rain, and I was intrigued.

Matt, however, lived in Pittsburgh, where he wrote for the *Pittsburgh Press*. On his way back there, he planned to visit his mother in Cambridge. My mother, who told me Matt was marriage material, suggested I leave the island and return to Cambridge, in hopes that Matt would call me there.

"Get off this island," were her exact words. "He's going to call you." I left. I went back to my rent-controlled apartment to wait for his call, and it came. My mother was right. I didn't always listen to everything she said. She could be super bossy, but by putting her thoughts into words, she confirmed what I had been hoping.

It didn't take long for me to know I wanted to marry Matt, a barrel-chested guy with a head of almost black hair, a straight Greek nose he inherited from his father, and dark brown eyes with a scar near his chin from when he was six and ran through a glass door after his sisters and babysitter, who were going to a part of town where he thought he could see dump trucks at a construction site.

That fall, I walked up Standish Street in Cambridge, alone, and said to the empty sidewalk, "You don't know it, Matt Brelis, but I'm going to marry you." I was twenty-nine and knew a good thing when I saw it. I had seen the alternatives. I tried to play it cool, however, when I was around him—something he later said I wasn't

good at. He knew I was ready for that ring. He picked up on my
eagerness and proposed six months later.

We married in the small white congregational church in
West Tisbury the following September. We had our reception in
Grandma's backyard in Lambert's Cove, underneath a big tent
overlooking the field and Vineyard Sound.

Maggie and Jay married in the field next door twenty-nine
years later, and I gave them a quilt of blues and oranges to represent the water surrounding the Vineyard and the sun rising and
setting.

But before I became proficient in quilt-making, I made Matt
one for a wedding present. That one almost didn't get made.

After Matt and I got engaged, I mentioned I wanted to give
him a quilt for his wedding present. Perhaps I said this over the
phone while he was in Pittsburgh and I was in Cambridge. Perhaps
we were together on a weekend visit.

Wherever we were, I remember what he said. "That's not a
present for me. That's a present for us."

The minute the words were out of his mouth, he tried to take
them back, but the words already hung in the air.

I was still a neophyte at quilting, but I enjoyed selecting fabric and patterns and then the whole process of putting it together
block by block, putting order to chaos.

Matt's quilt proved to be challenging. Queen-sized quilts were
different from baby quilts. I wasn't sure I had the ability or time,
but it was worth trying, even though he might not want it. I made
it without telling him. I worked on it during the week when we
were apart and put it in a closet when we were together on the
weekends. I chose the wedding chain pattern in cornflower blues
for the small squares and white for the large ones. I didn't yet know

how to quilt it together, so I tied it—knotting it over and over to keep the batting in place.

I worked feverishly up to the wedding day. I brought it to the Vineyard and laid it out on my grandmother's green rug in her green TV room. I purchased batting at the local quilting store, Heath Hen, in Vineyard Haven. Again, not knowing what I know now, I thought the batting looked thin, so I doubled it up—a big mistake, as it made the quilt heavy and hot—and started my knotting. Every spare minute I had during the week before the wedding, I sat on the floor knotting and tying floss through the quilt to hold it in place.

Two nights before our wedding, Matt and I went out to dinner at the Beach Plum Inn in Menemsha, which overlooked the harbor, with its fishing boats and pleasure yachts. It was just the two of us, where we could be alone to celebrate our upcoming life together.

I had gone to a jewelry store in Vineyard Haven that specialized in antique watches and bought him a handsome analog watch with numbers in the face encased in gold.

At dinner, he gave me a strand of pearls wrapped in paper from Bramhall & Dunn, a high-end home design store also in Vineyard Haven, to throw me off. A friend and neighbor in Lambert's Cove wrapped the present for him. The pearls matched the earrings he had given me as an engagement present. I handed him the box with the watch.

He looked at me, eyebrows furrowed. "Where's my quilt?" he asked.

"You said you didn't want it."

He looked like a little boy caught reading a book under the covers with his flashlight. He was so busted.

He loved the watch. He wore it for years, until, like the rest of the world, he started checking his iPhone for the time.

The following night, our families convened for the rehearsal dinner at Le Grenier, a French restaurant in Vineyard Haven. A huge collection of wine corks stood at attention on the windowsills. We took up half the restaurant. Our parents and stepparents were on their best behavior. There were no snide comments or side-eyes. As the evening progressed, friends and family made toast after toast to Matt and me. We returned to Le Grenier every summer for more than twenty-five years, to remember that evening, until the restaurant closed a few years before the pandemic.

I can preside in front of a classroom of students and teach, but standing up in a room full of people I know and love in order to make a toast made me swim with dizziness. But that night, I was ready to stand and toast Matt. Thirty-four years later, I can't remember what I said, but I do remember I told him I had something to show him how much I loved him.

My brother, Will, and my sister, Trina, went to the bathroom where we had hidden the quilt. When I signaled, they came and spread it out.

We call it the quilt that made Matt cry.

We slept under the heavy quilt for years, sweating and kicking it off in the middle of the night. When Maggie was about four, she colored on the quilt with my red lipstick. Although devastated at first, I realized the red simply added more story to the life of the quilt. And as time went on, the quilt showed its age, just like the weight around my stomach grew as my family expanded when Ellie, daughter number two, came into our lives.

Matt's quilt was also coming apart in many places, and holes appeared where the floss came undone and fell out. The pillow-casing technique doesn't protect the edges the same way binding does, and more holes and rips appeared.

Its wear-and-tear exposed itself, just like in my marriage the year we fought over how to load and unload a dishwasher. I balled it up sometime when my kids were in their preteens and I was tired of where my life was. My mother had died, my career was flatlining, and I ripped the back of the quilt from the top, intending to fix the holes and put it back together again.

But, it sat on the floor in a corner of our bedroom, reminding me to get a grip. Time went on, and my mother's death had less of a hold on me. Matt and I enjoyed our family life of soccer, church, and homework. I was engaged in my teaching, and Matt was wrapped up in reporting and editing at *The Boston Globe*. I found a way to write more, and the time came to celebrate that quilt again.

When I decided to fix Matt's wedding quilt, I knew I didn't have the skill or patience to mend all the torn pieces, so I took it to the Cambridge Quilt Shop, and there, Lynn took it on as a project. She found similar fabric to replace the pieces that had ripped, she mended the seams and holes, and even the lipstick is paler, but still there. I found material to bind it and a new back, and I took it to a woman who could actually quilt it together on her long arm quilting machine, instead of using the knotting and tying method. It was ready for Christmas.

Matt didn't cry this time when he opened it; he didn't even recognize it at first. He thought it was a new quilt. When he realized it was the same one, just repaired, he was flabbergasted. He quickly asked, "Is the lipstick still there?" He loved that lipstick.

It is back on our bed again. It doesn't fit the king-size bed we graduated to, but it accents our down comforter, and the dogs—who now sleep with us, instead of our long ago babies—love to nestle in it.

Matt and I always made it to the Vineyard in the summer, and in the early years of our marriage, we stayed at my grandmother's. When I miscarried my first pregnancy, we grieved and healed at Lambert's Cove in June, sleeping on a mattress in the living room as painters were busy on the second floor.

A year later, my mother and Dads set out to find their own place on the island, where they could be more independent and Dads could putter—he built stone walls, created a meadow, and kept the place running. They were in their late-fifties and early-sixties. I was thirty-three and pregnant with Maggie. They bought a developer's Cape Cod "spec" house in the Chilmark woods and modified it for their needs, adding a wing for visitors, a.k.a their children. By the time Maggie was five and Ellie was two, they had built an 800-square-foot guesthouse, where we stayed when we visited.

The girls and I took full advantage of their generosity. I was the only grown child with children and a flexible schedule, so we went to the island every summer, and Matt visited on weekends. We went to the beach when he came and sometimes had my parents, his sister's family (who also stayed on the Vineyard), and friends over for dinners. As my kids got older and my siblings built their own families and wanted to use the guesthouse, our time on the Vineyard diminished.

As young kids, Maggie and Ellie went to day camp in Chilmark in the mornings, where they played kickball, did arts and crafts, put on theater performances and learned to sail. I played tennis daily, with new friends or my mother and her friends, while the kids were busy at their summer program. After a lunch of egg salad sandwiches at home, we went to the beach with my mother. We spent an inordinate amount of time in the water. The girls jumped waves and learned to dive under them.

As they grew older, they worked at the day camp—in the snack bar, where Maggie met Jay, and as counselors responsible for the children they once were. We spent fewer afternoons at the beach as they hung out with friends or preferred to nap and read books.

With Spray in heat the summer of 2009, our Vineyard trip was in jeopardy. We didn't know it then, but Spray, like Splash, had her own idiosyncrasies, but they weren't as obnoxious. Unlike most bitches who go into heat (or season) twice a year, Spray went into heat every three or four months, which was tiring. I couldn't bring her to a place on the Vineyard where there weren't fences and I couldn't protect her.

Matt solved the problem by forgoing his weekend visits to the island. He and Spray stayed in Cambridge. While he missed us, he loved Spray and bonded even more with her. When the girls and I went home at the end of the summer, Matt and I jumped right back into our disagreement about breeding.

"See," I said. "See what a nightmare it was. The blood. The humping. The missed weekends."

He didn't flinch.

"Morg, just think how much fun it would be for all of us," he said, reminding me again of his childhood and his mother's dream. "Mom wanted to breed Charlotte, but we couldn't ever get it done," he said, remembering his big Newfoundland.

"It'll be scary. We don't know what we're doing. It'll be irresponsible. And guess who will be doing most of the work?" I asked. "I don't want to be a backyard breeder."

I didn't want to admit it, but I was beginning to come around. I was terrified of making a mistake, but Spray's temperament was so appealing, the thought of what her puppies might be like was exciting.

Bitches can't be bred until they are two, so if we went forward with breeding, the puppies would be born during Maggie's senior year. Instead of taking a family trip somewhere exciting in Europe during her final spring break (our original plan), we would be home raising puppies.

"Are you sure you're okay with this?" I asked at the wooden kitchen counter back in Cambridge one night. "We could go away or stay home with puppies."

"I don't want Spray to die," Ellie said, still worried about the process.

"She'll be fine, I promise," Matt said.

"Yes," said Maggie. "I'm totally okay with this. It'll be fun."

The learning curve was going to be steep. There was a lot to find out about breeding, and I wanted to make sure we did it the right way. There wasn't much time for me to learn it all. Maybe this project could distract me from obsessing about Maggie's impending departure from our family.

CHAPTER FIVE

In order to breed a dog properly, she needs a series of tests to determine whether she is genetically appropriate for breeding. To learn about these tests and the breeding process, our breeder, Sandy Nightingale, suggested I take Spray to Slade Veterinary Clinic in Framingham, Massachusetts, which specializes in reproductive health.

While I waited for my appointment, Sandy emailed me a photo of Brady, the stud dog she had found for us. He was also a product of one of her breedings, but with different parentage than Spray. Brady was named after then-Patriots quarterback Tom Brady. As an avid football family, dedicated to the Patriots, this matchup was perfect. Matt and Maggie were true diehard Pats fans. Matt had season tickets, and more often than not, he and Maggie went to the games. Ellie and I went to one game a year, usually in the early fall when the weather was still warm. We watched the rest of the season fastened to our seats in front of the TV.

Brady, like his namesake, was an appropriately commanding dog. Black, with a large white necklace, he stood up tall, with a big square head.

No longer just hypothetical cute fuzzballs, the puppies took shape and color in my mind. Sandy had warned me that Spray could "throw" a lot of white and possibly some brown (as Cocoa,

Spray's mom, was brown). I wasn't sure why this was critical. I didn't care. I loved Spray's unique color combo. The most common color for Portuguese water dogs, however, is black with some white markings. But, PWDs can be brown and white as well. For showing purposes, all colors are considered proper conformation of the breed, just as the two cuts—lion and retriever—are acceptable.

The retriever cut looks just like it sounds: even all the way around, like a retriever dog. The lion cut, however, is quite different. The back end of the dog is shaved to show their muscular hindquarters. They can also swim faster without so much hair, but it looks like they don't have pants on. PWDs have one of two coats. One is called "wavy," and it resembles ocean waves when it bounces as the dog runs. The second is "curly" and is just that, with tight curls like a standard poodle. Both can get matted easily and must be brushed and groomed regularly. We've had both types.

Despite the fact that we weren't planning on showing Spray or any of her pups, we wanted to be responsible, and we put Spray through all the tests required of PWD breeders.

Slade Veterinary Hospital looks nondescript from the outside. An old, shingled house in Framingham, inside it looked more like a vet's office. Two receptionists behind a big desk greeted me when I walked in onto the linoleum flooring. Photographs of litters and thank you cards from breeders covered the walls. The distinct smell of dog wafted through the waiting area.

Spray and I were called into a small examining room to wait for our vet: a blonde woman with her arm in a cast. She looked serious, like a high school biology teacher.

I sat on the floor petting Spray, trying to calm her as she paced back and forth. Before Dr. Serious gave the squirming Spray an internal exam, she handed me diagrams and printouts of articles

and up-to-date information on breeding. She explained how pro-
gesterone levels increased before ovulation, during which time
Spray returned to Slade's for daily blood tests. She told me about
estrogen, cornification (the thickening of the uterine wall) and the
different options for inseminating Spray.

We could choose natural insemination, which was the least
expensive method, but, the vet said with her eyes locked on mine,
Spray ran the risk of being injured during "the act." When dogs
mate, I learned, they lock onto each other and sometimes cannot
unlock, and it can be quite painful. A breeder can only wait it out.

We could also opt for artificial insemination, in which the
sperm is collected, spun, and injected into Spray. "This is more expensive, Morgan, but less risky," she said, "and the results will be
more or less guaranteed." Finally, confusing me completely, she said
we could go with the most certain and expensive method: surgically
implanting the sperm.

"I didn't know I was going to have options," I said, staring at
her, my mind racing. I needed to call Sandy. I couldn't make this
decision alone. Sandy calmly told me to choose AI, artificial insemination. It was what she had done, and it was the safest, most
effective and moderately affordable option.

I then had to decide between live and frozen sperm. Brady, our
stud dog, was local, so I chose live—Brady would go to the office to
contribute his sperm when the timing was right.

Each time Dr. Serious brought up a new topic, she gave me
a new handout, like I was back in science class, where I hadn't
excelled. This visit was making me feel like I had in high school:
dumb. I was lucky I wasn't being graded because I would've failed.
I was doomed. I nodded my head, looked her in the eye, hoped she
thought I was paying attention and prayed I'd be able to make sense

of the literature when I got home and had both time and Matt to look it over.

Matt didn't get as flustered as I did. He could decode scientific material. Perhaps his years as a journalist helped him decipher complicated information. With good eye contact, he calmly explained whatever it was I didn't understand. He didn't judge me when I didn't understand the national or international news. If I couldn't say a particular multisyllabic word—a carryover from my early years when I struggled with language—he repeated the word, broke it into the appropriate syllables and had me repeat it back. Then I could incorporate it into my speech or written work.

Sandy helped me too. Without her direction, I would have been completely lost, the way I am when I drive in the suburbs and my lack of directional ability kicks in. But Sandy was in Rhode Island, and I needed someone closer who could help me with the actual delivery, so I asked Laura N., my friend and neighbor, to be our midwife.

I had known Laura since Maggie and Laura's oldest, Alix, were in pre-K together. She was perfect for the job. She lived around the corner, she was a nurse practitioner, she wasn't easily upset, and she and her partner had bred their own Labradors eleven times by the time Matt and I thought of having puppies. If anyone could help me in the moment, it would be unflappable Laura. Years later, she and her partner had four litters during the pandemic. She was an expert.

As I began to tell friends what we were planning, I got an earful from a close friend one June night as I exited the Brattle Theater in Harvard Square.

Mervan Osborne, a former drama teacher in the kids' school, ran a two-week film camp every June. Maggie and Ellie had participated in Cinemaze as soon as they were eligible in fifth grade. Mervan shot on location all over Boston, edited the film, and then rented out the Brattle Theater to premiere it for family and friends. Both Maggie and Ellie were actors. Both entered the acting and entertainment world as young adults post-college.

Mervan was a friend, as well as the kids' film director, and one day when he was visiting us, he met Spray (when she was just a puppy) and was smitten. "I want one of her puppies," he said. "I'll name it Sparky." We hadn't even decided we were going forward with the breeding. He was way ahead of us.

As people left *The Man with the Plutonium Legs*, a film loosely based on *The Usual Suspects*, Mervan turned to me. "I can't wait for a puppy," he said as he put his arm around me.

"Don't hold your breath," I said. "It's a long process. There's a lot to do."

Susie, standing next to me, turned. "You're not breeding your dog, are you? Do you know how many dogs in shelters need homes? You shouldn't add to the problem."

I turned my face like she had slapped it and backed away.

I did agree with her. I knew tons of people, including my siblings, who rescued dogs, but we couldn't because of the allergies in our family. There were other families out there like ours who wanted a puppy. I was taking on a lot by agreeing to breed Spray, and I was still a little reluctant. This dressing down didn't help.

Mervan's wife, Lucy, then put her arm around me and said, "We still want one of Spray's puppies."

I worried, constantly. Were my friends and family going to assume I had completely lost my mind? Would I be a responsible breeder? What about Spray's health and the health of her puppies? Could I handle squeezing all this into our already busy schedules? Would we be able to find homes for the puppies?

When I asked Sandy what she liked about breeding, she said the best part was giving puppies to families—that gave her great joy. "Breeding is fraught with trouble, and you shouldn't go into it lightly," she warned. "Bitches get sick, puppies die in birth, and you are forever tied to the puppies you send out into the world." She was right.

We went to New Hampshire at the end of August to celebrate Labor Day and Matt's birthday. It had been another summer of Spray being in heat and Matt missing the Vineyard. In New Hampshire, we knew no one (unlike on the Vineyard, where we were surrounded by family and friends), so we just focused on being together with the four of us.

We stayed at the rustic camp in Sandwich, near Squam Lake, that Matt and his three older sisters inherited from their aunt and uncle. The camp was built in the early 1900s on rock pillars, without a basement. It was a seasonal house—the uninsulated wooden walls were still their natural dark brown. The small windows didn't let in much light. For someone who needs light to feel good (I even have a light box in my home office), the dark rusticity could feel cramped, oppressive, and depressing. But Matt loved it, and I enjoyed being alone with our kids. I didn't worry about anyone else's agenda; it was just Splash, Spray and the four of us.

As we sat by the fire in the large stone fireplace one night—after roasting and burning marshmallows—Maggie braided Ellie's long, light brown hair, I realized it could be the last time they did this. The next fall, Maggie would be in college, somewhere, and even if we came to Squam, Ellie would be alone. The days of the four of us were numbered.

We were entering a year of lasts. Just like I had recorded all her firsts in a baby journal, I was now starting to note Maggie's lasts—her last high school field hockey game, her last high school play, the last year the four of us ate dinner at the kitchen counter, the last time we would go to church together, the last time we'd squish on the couch to watch a movie.

I wasn't ready.

But after Ellie and I combed Keepsake Quilting for fabric for Maggie's quilt, I figured concentrating on the sewing would take the focus off the real adventure ahead—Maggie leaving home.

In early September, when the weather was still warm, we drove back to Rhode Island to meet Brady, Spray's intended. This time, we knew where we were going. We recognized the familiar landmarks of the bay at the border between Massachusetts and Rhode Island. Ellie wasn't worried about the destination; she was excited about meeting Brady. Maggie and Ellie took turns holding Spray in their laps in the back seat.

When we arrived, the Nightingales escorted us through the breezeway out to the back deck, where they offered us drinks and cookies at a round table with an umbrella raised to shelter us from the sun. Then Brady and his owner, Sam, showed up. His photograph didn't do him justice. A curly PWD two years Spray's senior, he looked like his photo—his body and the top of his large square head were black, while his chest and scarf were white. Any offspring from Spray and Brady were destined to be stunning.

Brady and Spray sniffed each other. Once we determined they were going to behave, we dropped the leashes and let them explore the back deck and yard, which included a play area covered in pea stones for dogs to romp in. They followed each other around, dragging their leashes, oblivious to the humans drinking iced tea and eating cookies.

We discussed the logistics of the actual insemination and the stud fee, which was only $1,500 because Brady hadn't fathered a litter yet. By the time we went through with the insemination, however, his services cost more, as he had fathered another litter and his value increased by progeny of known quality.

Driving back from Rhode Island, we bounced around in the car. We were really going through with this. We had a stud dog. We had Spray. We were going to have a litter of puppies. I didn't know whether to laugh because we were taking on a great adventure, or cry because we were crazy.

Maggie was the starting goalie for the varsity field hockey team at her high school.

When we weren't encouraging her to write her college essay, which she hadn't done over the summer like we had suggested, Matt and I were at her games cheering the team on from the sidelines.

Maggie loved being a goalie, the last wall of defense, and I was proud of her. Still, I was anxious watching her games. My stomach clenched when the ball got near her end of the field. "Get it out!" I yelled, and I paced a lot. I hated seeing a ball sail into her goal and then watching Maggie's reaction.

She was often better at shaking off the goals than me. Her body language always told me how she was feeling. When she rounded her shoulders and dragged her stick a little, she didn't feel good. I knew she thought she could or should have stopped the goal. If she took the ball and shot it down the field with her stick, then she was pissed but okay. She knew the goal had been a good one. Over the years, she learned to accept the good goals and move on and push herself to play better when she let in a bad goal. She was also able to recognize what was her responsibility and what was her defense's.

Perhaps these lessons on the field would transfer to life lessons off the field. Maybe when the college acceptances and rejections started coming in, she'd be able to shake them off as well. I wasn't convinced, though, as Maggie, like her dad, is ultracompetitive. They thrive on winning (and on watching the Patriots win as well), whereas Ellie and I just don't care. Even though I play tennis and board games, I generally feel bad when I'm beating someone at a game and often make a mistake to let the other person have the upper hand—not a useful habit to have when playing games of any sort.

Matt went to as many of Maggie's field hockey games as possible, leaving work early if he could, and the parents, players and coaches always knew when he was there, as he bellowed from the sidelines, "Go Knights!" "Go Blue!" He didn't need a megaphone. His deep voice resonated. I fell in love with his voice when we started dating. If the games were on the weekend, we often brought Spray. She was so well-behaved and sweet, a welcome addition to the fans.

Maggie wanted to play field hockey in college, which added another dimension to the application process. She went to several summer camps at different colleges—large and small—Division I and Division III—such as Yale, Amherst, BC, and Vassar. She decided to play for a Division III school, where she could play field hockey, but unlike a Division I school, she wouldn't have to play year-round. She would have time for her other interests, like film.

At home, Maggie immersed herself in homework, but she still hadn't written her college essay. She spent a lot of time behind her closed door, where the floor was littered with clothes and books. I hoped she was working on the essay, but given how Maggie liked to procrastinate, I worried she wasn't. Years later, as a young adult, Maggie was diagnosed with ADD, which made so much sense. Had I figured that out sooner, maybe she would have had an easier time with deadlines.

Our kitchen counter was covered with dishes for dinner at one end and papers and books at the other. Splash lay directly underneath Maggie, and Ellie and Spray sat in the armchair in the adjoining living room, while we ate our dinner and tried hard not to talk about college. The college counselors had suggested setting aside one day a week as the college day. That was great in theory, but hard to practice as college was on our minds all the time, especially when Matt and I had no idea if Maggie was making any headway on her applications.

"Maggie, making any progress on those applications?" I might have asked between bites of green beans.

"Oh no," Ellie sighed. College was three years off for her.

Maggie cut me off, "Yup," shaking her head of thick, dark brown hair.

"How's it going?" Matt followed up.

"Fine."

Dinner then proceeded in silence, unless one of us brought up what we would do for the weekend. I hate confrontation, so I left Maggie alone to stew in her misery, knowing it would catch up with her soon.

"You know," Matt said one night. "My mother grounded me when I had to do my applications, so if you don't get yours done, the same thing will happen. We'll ground you."

"Yup," Maggie acknowledged.

When we did the dishes after dinner, Spray jumped from her chair and hung out by the dishwasher, hoping crumbs would fall from the plates as they got passed around. The girls handed their dirty dishes to us and disappeared as fast as they could, to avoid any more college talk.

CHAPTER SIX

As Maggie filled out her college applications behind her closed door, the American Kennel Club returned Spray's registration form—I had filled it out incorrectly, listing us as joint owners with the Nightingales, instead of sole owners. The terms confused me. Time to start over, slowing the whole process down. Spray was due to go into heat in November, and we were required to have the AKC registration finalized before we could do the testing. Time was running out.

My classroom and students were my sole distraction. No matter how many papers I had to correct, how much I had to prepare for my classes, once I was in a classroom with my students, everything else in my life dropped away. There was only me and my students talking about writing—whether we were discussing revision strategies or critiquing a student essay—the only thing I worried about was whether my students were engaged and learning.

I was an adjunct faculty member at Emerson, where I had completed my MA in Professional Writing and Publishing, graduating cum laude. While I had also held brief stints at the Harvard Extension School, University of Pittsburgh, and Boston University, I always returned to Emerson because it attracted inquisitive and focused students. I taught the two subjects I enjoyed and excelled at: magazine writing and creative nonfiction. Both fell under the jurisdiction of the Writing, Literature, and Publishing Department.

Being an adjunct is challenging. I had no access to departmental decisions, and while there were examples of adjuncts who became term or full-time professors, they were few. Some of the full-time faculty walked by the adjuncts as though walking through ghosts. I had applied twice for a full-time deal, but without a book to my name, I couldn't cross the line in the sand that washed away with every wave.

Once in the classroom, however, I forgot about my adjunct position and the dead end. I even forgot about the inequity of pay between adjuncts and full-timers. I combined my teaching with freelancing for the *Globe*, *The Boston Parents Paper*, some alumni magazines, and other publications. Luckily, Matt had good benefits at *The Boston Globe*, and later as Director of Communications at Massport, the organization that owns and operates Logan Airport, Hanscom Field, the cruise and container terminals in the Port of Boston, and real estate holdings.

I often thought about not teaching—less time correcting papers and prepping for class—but I never left. I adored the students. I loved reading their work and getting to know them through their writing. My world was broadened by learning about different cultures, jobs, the LGBTQ world, and music. I never knew from semester to semester what would grab me. I got jazzed as my students engaged with their own work and their peers' work. It was exciting. Every semester was stimulating.

The AKC paperwork had been approved, and I took Spray to Slade Veterinary so often she knew where we were when I turned the corner into the driveway. As soon as I parked the car, Spray, surprisingly, jumped out and pulled on her leash, leading me up the ramp to the front of the building and into the waiting area. Even at her regular vet, she led me up the path and into the office. She was always happy.

Inside Slade, a vet tech called "Spray?" and took the leash from me. Spray walked off, turning her head to look back at me. Was she wondering why I wasn't going with her? Once the day's tests—X-rays of her hips and elbows or blood tests—were complete, Spray returned to me. She leapt in joy when she saw me.

We signed the stud contract and paid the rest of the fee—$1000. The bitch Brady had inseminated was carrying eleven puppies. Sandy reassured me that was most unusual. While the stud determines the puppies' gender, the bitch determines the size of the litter, and Spray most likely was carrying about seven, like her mother.

I filed this information away in the back of my brain, knowing I would need it later. I operated on a need-to-know basis. The minute I started to take in too much, I shut down. I've always learned best this way. I learn by doing. I could read a whole instruction manual and still not know how a TV remote worked. I had to hold it in my hand to fully understand how it operated.

Spray continued to be tested; she needed an ophthalmology evaluation, for which she went to an eye doctor an hour south of Boston. She also needed DNA tests. For these, we swabbed the inside of her mouth and put the swabbing stick in a package and mailed it to the testing site.

Spray passed all her tests and was ready for breeding.

By the end of October, Maggie knew where she was going to apply and wasn't going to be swayed by her parents. We hoped she would apply early decision to Vassar. Not only because Matt and I had gone there, but also, the field hockey coach wanted her and could put a chit in for her at admissions if she applied early, but not during regular admissions time. Matt and I decided it was a great fit, but Maggie dug her heels in. She didn't love the place. "It reminds me of a boarding school," she repeatedly told us. She wanted options; she didn't want to be locked into one place.

By November 15, Maggie's essay still wasn't done, and Spray still hadn't gone into heat. The one time I wanted Spray to be on time, she wasn't. Thanksgiving was creeping up on us, and we had planned to go to the Vineyard to join Dads, my sister (Trina), and my brother (Will). I didn't want to eat my turkey at Slade Veterinary.

Whenever I worried about Spray and the next steps in breeding, I phoned or emailed Sandy, and she calmed me down. Too bad she couldn't do the same thing with Maggie and her applications. Maggie's stress radiated off her like heat waves from hot pavement. She waited until the last possible moment before the early action deadline to send her applications to two Scottish schools and the University of Vermont. She had fallen in love with Scotland when she traveled to Iona, an island off the coast, with her church youth group.

The night before early action deadlines for the first round of applications, she slithered out from her room and sat at the kitchen counter, where she glared at Matt and me as she filled out her forms. With great fanfare, she hit the send button, and I took a picture of her. She still had more applications to go, but she had made a big dent in the process.

Right before Thanksgiving, Spray went into heat. Her timing wasn't ideal. After more blood tests, the vets and Sandy calculated that she would be most fertile the day after Thanksgiving. So, we made it to the Vineyard for some quick turkey, but there wasn't time for a weekend of walks on the beach or holiday shopping at the annual craft fair, which Matt and Will called the "Crap Fair." We quickly zipped up our still-packed bags, leashed the dogs, and returned early Friday morning. Matt went straight to the airport, where he worked, and after dropping the girls and Splash at home, I took my car and drove to Framingham, where I met up with Sandy and Jim, Diane, Sam, and Brady.

We sat in the waiting area watching Brady strain at his leash, trying to get to Spray. He was like a frat boy at a dance. I was nervous and awkward. I knew Sandy and Jim and appreciated them being there for everyone's best interest, but I was almost shy around Diane and Sam. It felt a little like a blind date, and I wasn't sure what to say. "Oh look, Brady looks really excited about donating sperm!" Nope, how about, "I can't wait to find out if Spray gets pregnant!"

A friendly doctor arrived on the scene and took Brady and Sam into one of the examining rooms to "collect" the sperm. One of the vet techs followed with Spray. When they were finished with Brady, they called me into another room down the hall, where I found Spray in a corral-like pen, on a ramp with her head pointed toward the bottom and her rump raised higher.

The doctors spun the sperm in a machine to make it more concentrated and therefore stronger. Then, using a syringe, they injected it into Spray. The vet then set a timer and "feathered" Spray, placing her gloved fingers inside Spray to make sure the sperm reached her cervix.

Spray, much to my surprise, didn't seem as disturbed by what seemed to me a violation to her body. She stood stoically in the pen and occasionally looked over at me with a when-are-we-going-to-be-done look on her face.

"Good dog, Spray," I said. "You're such a good dog." I was so out of my comfort zone in the tiny room, but I didn't want Spray to pick up on any of my feelings, so I stroked her and cooed to her. "I love you. Good dog," I repeated.

When the timer went off, I took Spray from the room. Dr. Friendly said there wasn't any reason to think the procedure hadn't worked, and Spray should deliver sixty-three days later, in January. To hedge our bets, however, the vets recommended we bring Spray back for another round of insemination in two days. Oh goody.

The next time, it was just Spray, Brady, Matt, Sam, and me.

When Dr. Friendly came out to the waiting area to get the dogs, she asked who had helped last time. When she realized Matt hadn't been around at all, she smiled and said, "Oh, you. You come with me."

Matt and Spray followed Brady and Sam back to the examining rooms, leaving me alone in the waiting area to flip through books about dogs.

Later, Matt shared what had happened so I, too, could enjoy the gory details. "They used Spray as a tease for Brady. But she just sat down. She didn't want anything to do with it," he said. "Then the doc turns to me and says, 'Get her to stand. You know you men,' she laughed, 'you like your visuals.' Poor Spray. So, I made her stand, and Brady did what he had to, and they collected his stuff."

Matt didn't really like the feathering part either. "I felt so bad for her, standing there with this woman's fingers inside of her," he said.

But once it was over and done, Spray didn't seem any different.

She went back to being Spray. She danced in circles, turning around and around in place when excited, especially when we came home at the end of the day or when we let Splash and her out into the backyard. She lay on the back cushions of our couch, wrestled with Splash, and sat in her armchair. There were no more road trips, blood tests, or invasive procedures. It was now time to wait and see.

As time went on, Spray slowed down. While she never looked huge, and strangers on the street didn't always believe us when we said she was pregnant, her abdomen was firm and compressed, the way brown sugar is packed. She took to sitting in her chair without moving.

On December 22, a month after the insemination—in the midst of my final papers, grades, and Christmas shopping—Ellie and I took Spray back to Framingham for an ultrasound to confirm the pregnancy. Although it wouldn't be definitive, the ultrasound would give us a sense of how many puppies she was carrying.

The vet tech shaved Spray's tummy, laid her in a cradle-like contraption with her stomach facing up, and put jelly on her belly. I could almost feel the cold blob against my skin, from when I had ultrasounds during my pregnancies with the girls. The tech took the wand and rolled it over Spray's abdomen.

There they were, the puppies—or what we were told were puppies—on the screen. They looked like lima beans, all five of them. The vet printed out photos for us to put on our refrigerator at home and reminded me that ultrasounds were unreliable. There could be more pups, or one could be reabsorbed between the ultrasound and delivery. We wouldn't know for sure how many lima beans she was carrying until a final X-ray a few days before the pups were due in late January. Unlike humans, dogs always give birth on their actual due date.

One day before winter break, I was in my cubicle at Emerson, correcting papers when my phone chimed.

I picked up my cellphone and hit the answer button. "Hi, Mags, what's up?"

"I heard. I got into Glasgow!"

"Oh my God!"

"Now I know I'm going to college," she practically yelled. I could hear her smiling.

Shortly after that, she learned she had been admitted early to the University of Vermont with some scholarship assistance, but she still wasn't ready to commit anywhere. She needed to finish her applications, which would make our winter break stressful. Her birthday—five days after Christmas—usually extended our holiday season. But this year, it too was going to be sheathed in stress.

Maggie did finish the rest of her applications during winter break because we grounded her, just like we said. Even during a snowstorm, when her boyfriend Jay—who lived forty minutes west of Cambridge—and Ellie went outside for a snowball fight with the neighbors, we kept Maggie inside, except for a quick, cold ten-minute break.

"Spray's mom?" called the vet tech from across the waiting room at Slade. She waved at me to follow her into the room where Spray had been inseminated in November. In January, she was being X-rayed to verify how many pups she was carrying.

Spray's X-ray was displayed on a large screen. I didn't know what I was looking at. "Each puppy," Dr. Friendly explained, "grows in its individual sac." I nodded. For female dogs, the uterus has two long arms, called *horns*, where the puppies grow like links on a chain. During birth, they take turns sliding down the horns and depositing themselves in the uterus before coming through the birth canal and out into the world.

After Dr. Friendly showed me one puppy sac, she pointed to each sac and counted. She got to five and kept counting. She counted to seven, and I nodded my head again, having assumed Spray would have more than the five on the original ultrasound.

But Dr. Friendly didn't stop at seven, the number I had banked on. "Eight." She pointed. I looked from Dr. Friendly to the vet tech. "Nine." She pointed. "Ten." She pointed. My mouth dropped open in a way that only happens in cartoons.

"There might be an eleventh in there," she added, "but we can't tell." She indicated an ambiguous shape high up on the screen.

I covered my mouth with my hand and stood still. I had nothing to say. Spray had ten puppies, chockablock inside her. That might explain her exceptionally hard stomach and why she didn't circle dance anymore. "Oh," I managed.

"Yes," Dr. Friendly said, "ten."

The vet tech told me to get Spray and follow her out to the reception area. There, I stood in a daze as she inundated me with information on the care Spray would need until she gave birth. I nodded my head a lot, as though I was following what she was saying. I shouldn't overfeed her. *Ten.* She would want only small meals spaced out during the day. *Ten.* I should give her a lot of water. *Ten.*

Both the vet and the tech recommended that Spray have a C-section, for safety reasons, because her litter was so large. Multiple hands would be available to pull the puppies out at the same time, and they could make sure each was healthy. It would also keep Spray from going into inertia and stalling out during the birthing process, which had happened to her mother. Puppies die that way. In the meantime, Spray also needed more blood work to help narrow down the time of her delivery.

I stood there, nodding. What I wondered but didn't say: *Ten fucking puppies?*

The idea of a C-section scared me, but the idea of dead puppies and/or a dead Spray-dog terrified me even more. I nodded my head once more, prayed I had retained some of what they were telling me and stumbled out of the office with Spray.

I stood in the parking lot and, before I even put Spray in the car, I texted Matt, Maggie, and Ellie one word: *TEN.*

I was going to be a nursemaid to ten puppies. We were going to have to clean up after ten puppies. We were going to have to find homes for ten puppies.

Ten. Really? Ten?

After the shock wore off and the fear subsided, I called my two mentors, Laura N. and Sandy. Laura, who used less medical intervention in her breeding experiences, thought Spray would be fine and could deliver the puppies on her own. Sandy, who had watched Cocoa experience inertia and lose two puppies, encouraged me to listen to Dr. Friendly.

Because Matt and I were new breeders, we decided to rely on medical technology. This seemed safer. I was afraid of dead puppies. If the experts at Slade thought a Cesarean would eliminate the risk to Spray and her pups, I was in, regardless of the additional $2,000.

Even experienced breeders are sad when puppies don't make it. Some breeders let natural selection take its toll—they won't work to save a weak puppy, knowing that vulnerable, little dogs often struggle to survive in the world and may die anyway, sometimes weeks later.

Other breeders go to extremes, even bottle-feeding the weakest and smallest puppies, trying to give them the boost they need until they are strong enough to keep going on their own. If fate dealt us a sick puppy, I'd fall in the second camp. I'm not a fan of death.

Common myth has it that the runt of the litter—the smallest and therefore weakest puppy—is the last born. Not so. The runt is determined by the puppies' locations in the mom's horns, which in turn determines their access to nutrients. The one who gets the fewest nutrients is the smallest, a.k.a. the runt.

Sandy and Jim had stopped breeding because they couldn't stand the pain that came with the process. Everything had gone well with their bitch Squiggy's first two litters. She had five pups the first time and seven the second. The third time, however, was catastrophic, Sandy told me. Squiggy went into labor early, and they used terbutaline—a medication that helps with asthma but also delays labor. Jim and Sandy brought her to the vet's, where they could monitor her more closely. There, they were told to go get some coffee before her scheduled Cesarean.

Sandy remembered returning to find a vet tech running down the hall with a pup in her hand. She told them to follow her. "We passed Squiggy on the operating table, all opened up with blood everywhere," Sandy said. Two vet techs were working on eight puppies, trying to get the mucus out of their airways so they could breathe. They lost three of the eight.

"It is something I will never forget and makes me so sad to this day," Sandy said.

After Cocoa, Spray's mom, had two stillborn pups in Spray's litter, Sandy couldn't do it anymore. "I'm just not cut out for all the terrible things that can go wrong with either the mother or the pups," she said. So, when we decided to breed Spray, they made a trip to

Cambridge to give us their whelping box and a huge Rubbermaid container full of blankets and soft lamb wool throws for the puppies to lie on. We figured if all went well, maybe we'd do it again.

When Dr. Friendly showed me Spray's X-ray, she explained how C-sections worked. Ten pairs of hands would grab all ten puppies the minute she opened Spray. A warming tray would be nearby with a heat lamp for them to snuggle under, and when Spray was stitched up, the pups could suckle on her.

Spray's C-section was scheduled for late Monday morning, three days away.

The office called later to say we needed to move the surgery up to first thing Monday morning. Spray's blood work indicated she might go into labor even earlier. We were to give her some terbutaline to stop the labor process.

Laura N. visited on Sunday evening and noticed that Spray was panting a lot. "Has she been rooting at all? In a corner anywhere?" she asked. "Watch her. If she starts digging or nesting in a corner, she will be ready to deliver."

What the hey?

I hoped the pups would be safely delivered by C-section the next morning. No dead puppies.

I went to bed on the third floor with Maggie and Ellie, and Matt slept with Spray on the big, brown couch in the back room on the first floor. Spray usually slept with us, often on Matt's chest just like our babies had, but she wasn't moving from the back room—maybe she was nesting—and Matt wanted to be sure someone was with her if she did go into labor.

We set our alarms for six a.m. to get to Slade for the seven a.m. procedure and went to bed.

CHAPTER SEVEN

"Morgan!" Matt's scream from the first floor reached the third floor and woke me up. "It's happening! I think it's dead."

"No." I leapt from my bed, ran past the girls' bedrooms, and charged downstairs.

I arrived in the back room, the coldest room in our house at the end of January, and found Matt holding a puppy in one hand, while Spray lay on the gray carpet at his feet.

"I think it's dead," Matt said again. He did not look overjoyed with the birth of this puppy. He stared at me as though I had an answer.

I didn't. I was going to kill Matt for coming up with this crazy idea, and now we had a dead puppy. This wasn't happening. My nightmare was coming to life.

Upstairs, Ellie had run into Maggie's room, screaming, "Maggie, Maggie! All the puppies are dead."

Maggie jolted awake, worried she had slept through her chemistry exam. Once she realized it was still hours away, she shifted her worry to the puppies.

The girls ran downstairs in their pajamas. Ellie stopped on the second floor. She had no interest in seeing dead puppies. She would wait it out. Maggie joined us. It was 3:30 in the morning, and we looked at each other, not sure what to do.

We weren't supposed to be alone. We had made our plans carefully to be either with Laura or a vet. Our plans were toast.

"Call someone," Matt barked.

When he had checked on Spray at one a.m., all was fine, he told me. But when he woke up again, Spray was licking something on his stomach—a puppy sac. Matt didn't know how long the puppy had been lying on top of him. He tore open the sac and then yelled for me.

I called Laura and the vet tech from Slade. Laura had been right. Spray wasn't waiting.

Laura told us to use a bulb syringe to suction the mucus out of the puppy's mouth, but I hadn't had one of those in the house since the kids were little. Almost immediately, she told us later, she turned to her partner and said, "That puppy is going to die."

The vet tech answered her phone and promptly hung up. "I wasn't wearing my glasses, and I can't hear or see without them. I was confused," she said. "How's Spray?"

"Spray's fine," I said. Spray sighed. She was unfazed by all the activity around her. I told her about the puppy.

"Morgan, tell Matt to hold the puppy in the palm of his hand, cover it with a towel and gently swing the puppy towards him from his shoulder down to his knees to clear its lungs." Before I could repeat the message, Matt was doing it.

"How'd you know to do that?" I asked.

"All that reading material you gave me," he answered and smiled. The puppy opened its mouth and peeped.

"Looks like the bitch is going to do it herself," the tech said and hung up.

The puppy breathed. I breathed.

The puppy lived. I let Matt live.

Ellie ran downstairs to join us.

We all stood there, looking at the puppy and then at each other. The pup was a white male with brown spots. His coat was slicked back, and he looked more like a mouse than a dog.

The girls cooed over him, but I wasn't sure he was that cute.

Spray paced around Matt's feet, until he leaned down and put the puppy under her nose so she could smell him. Then Matt laid him in the whelping box with a heating pad. He was very alone in the big box the Nightingales had given us. We hoped Spray would follow him and give birth to the rest of the puppies in there.

Whelping boxes are large wooden boxes in which the mother dog, or dam, can lie down to give birth, nurse and sleep with her pups. They have little shelves on the sides to keep the momma dog from rolling over on the puppies. Since Sandy had given us their whelping box, Spray was now going to give birth in the same box in which she had been birthed.

Except, she didn't want to get in the box.

I looked down the hallway and saw Laura standing on the other side of the glass oval in our front door. I could do this with Laura. We would be in capable hands. I couldn't believe she had come to us in the middle of the night. I took a deep breath. I could do this now.

Our urging finally got Spray to step into the whelping box, but instead of lying down with the puppy, she picked him up by the scruff of his neck and tried to deposit him outside the box.

I freaked.

"No, Spray, no. Put the puppy back," I almost yelled. I've been told repeatedly that my voice carries quite a distance. It's loud.

Maggie and Ellie joined in. "Spray, no," they chorused. "No, Spray."

Laura turned to me. "Morg, she thinks she did something bad, like she pooped. If you remain calm, she'll be calm. She doesn't want to be in the box. Are you okay if she gives birth on the rug?"

Whatever. My shoulders caved in.

"I'll be calm," I said and sank down on the floor next to Spray. I leaned against the couch. Even half asleep, Laura, with her cropped gray hair, was commanding.

Spray trusted me. She probably wanted all of us close to her. Bitches wouldn't let their loved ones out of their sight when they were birthing. We weren't planning on leaving her.

Despite the chaos in my house and my overcommitted life, when I needed to be calm, I was the coolest person going, the person you wanted to have in a crisis.

In 1997, a police officer called to tell me that Matt had gone into shock while tailgating at a Patriots game, and they didn't know if he was going to make it. I was composed on the phone, asking the pertinent questions about what the paramedics were doing to revive him.

"Are they giving him epinephrine? Steroids?" I asked the cop.

"I don't know. They're working on him," he answered.

I didn't flip out as I left a five-year-old and a two-year-old with a friend and drove from Cambridge to Foxboro—thirty-five miles, or fifty minutes—without knowing what I would find when I got there. I didn't own a cellphone.

When I walked into the hospital's ER, the nurse at check-in said, "You look worse than he did." That was enough for me. Matt was okay.

I always fell apart the day after a close call. Then I thought about what could have transpired and how lucky our family was.

Spray's early-morning labor was no different. She needed me, and I was there for her, the way I was there for Matt or the girls in a crisis, the way Matt had been there for me when I was in labor. I sat on the rug next to Spray and told her over and over what a good girl she was.

Watching Spray labor took me to a place I hadn't expected to go: nineteen years back in time, to five days after Christmas, when Matt and I had just moved into our new house. He was about to return to work after taking the week off. He was anxious about going back to his job, and he'd enjoyed a few glasses of wine to ease his nerves. Neither of us had planned on Maggie arriving a week early or me going into labor late on a Sunday night. But after eating a large dinner of leftover Christmas turkey, I didn't feel well. By the end of the evening, I knew what was happening.

By midnight, we were in the delivery room, and whenever Matt looked like he was about to fall asleep, I slugged him in the arm. "Don't you leave me!" I yelled.

He didn't. He roused himself and stayed awake all night.

As Matt likes to remind me, I also hollered for "the man with the fucking needle," desperate for the epidural to ease my pain, despite the doctor's warnings that the shot could cause paralysis or even cause death. I didn't care.

Matt stood by me when my epidural was injected, he held my hand and gave me ice chips, he encouraged me along the way. My delivery was a team effort.

I petted Spray and rubbed her side. "Good dog, Spray-Spray. I love you," I repeated.

Although we hadn't been prepared for a home birth, when Laura asked for blankets and towels, we had plenty. We quickly improvised a smaller, cozier whelping box, using a laundry basket with blankets and a warming disc—a round, plastic orb you microwave—and placed the puppies into that as each was born.

By almost four a.m., we relaxed a little. The puppy was alive, and Spray was resting.

Matt made a second attempt at making coffee. It was much better than the coffee Maggie had offered us earlier. Trying to be helpful, she volunteered to make Laura, Matt, and me coffee. She had never done this before, which became evident when she handed us brown water to drink. We stayed together for the next six hours, while Spray labored without any of the coaching or classes I'd had when I gave birth to Maggie, without watching any videos or listening to any lectures on breathing techniques. What she was doing was instinctual. While some bitches pace and squat through labor, Spray lay down and gently pushed each puppy out, making the birthing process look so easy.

Puppies don't necessarily come evenly spaced every two hours, and Spray's came at irregular intervals, so it was important for us to watch her carefully. Spray's stomach began to contract somewhere between half an hour and two hours after each puppy. If I put my hand on her abdomen, I could feel the next puppy move along the birth canal until her vulva widened and the puppy—inside a sac stretched like a thin stocking over its head—slipped into Laura's hands.

Laura either tore the sac open or held it out to Spray so she could open it with her teeth. Then Laura cut the umbilical cord with nail clippers and made sure the puppy was breathing. She held each puppy in her hand, wiped its body down with a towel, flipped it over and said, "boy" or "girl." She said "boy" six times (Matt had identified the first as a boy) and "girl" three times.

Most of our prospective buyers wanted females, knowing they tend to be a bit less rambunctious and more independent, although PWDs are known to attach themselves to their humans, following

them into the bathroom even. We had already committed one female to Mervan and we wanted to keep one for ourselves, which
meant we only had one available female—not a great situation.

I wondered what was going through Spray's mind. I got pregnant
by choice, and it was the best thing I've ever done—having my two
daughters, even though I hadn't wanted children. I didn't want to
harm my children somehow, the way I had been hurt. I didn't trust
that friends and family wouldn't desert me. I was insecure about my
life choices. My parents' divorce in the sixties had felt like waves
crashing on the beach. I didn't know which ones would knock me
down and which ones would lap at my feet. I didn't want anyone to
go through the feelings of abandonment that I had.

But did Spray want puppies? She didn't have a choice. Did she
worry about being a good mom? Or would she be pissed off with
her ten children?

Matt was upset when we were first married, and I told him I
didn't want children. This wasn't in his plan. He watched me play
with my goddaughter and his nieces and saw what he thought was
a good mother in the making. What he didn't understand was that
hanging out with other people's offspring was fun partly because I
could be the cool, kooky relative, and then I could walk away at the
end of the day.

When we started trying, I became pregnant faster than we had
anticipated, but I remained anxious about being a mother, worried
about the mistakes I would make, terrified of sending a child to the
therapist's couch. Wasn't I supposed to be giddy with excitement?

Just seven weeks in, and just as I was beginning to get used to
the idea, the pregnancy ended at a friend's wedding in Chicago. I

just wanted to go home, get into bed and cry. I hadn't realized how much I did want a baby.

Instead of flying back to Boston, I was taken by ambulance from O'Hare—where we were trying to get on a flight home—to nearby Resurrection Hospital, where doctors performed a D&C to remove any remaining fetal matter. I stayed overnight on the maternity ward after my surgery, listening to new babies cry as their mothers and fathers answered with exclamations of delight.

I sobbed for the child I would never know, convinced my ambivalence had caused the miscarriage. I cried when a social worker told Matt and me, "Name it. Pray to it."

"I want my baby," I said to Matt, between bursts of tears.

Matt had often challenged me by playing the *"Who's This?"* game when music played on the radio. I wasn't very good. He excelled. In the recovery room, "Keep Me Hanging On" played in the background. I looked up from my bed at Matt. "Matt, who's this?" He smiled down at me. "The Supremes."

Almost a year later, after Matt's mom died of cancer at sixty-one—another tragic loss—I became pregnant with the baby who turned out to be Maggie. I spent the early part of the pregnancy paranoid something bad might happen again, and I worried throughout the rest of the pregnancy about what kind of mother I was going to be.

Three years later, pregnant with Ellie, I wasn't quite as anxious. No matter what pain the pregnancy or childbirth brought, no matter what I didn't know about parenting multiple children, I knew for sure we would end up with a fabulous baby, an adorable permanent member of our lives. Our family would be complete. While we always talked about having a third, it wasn't to be.

I learned over the years that I would make my own mistakes

parenting my daughters. Staying in a committed relationship with Matt and staying put in our house in Cambridge gave my daughters the stability I wanted, but there were other areas where I failed—my moods were unpredictable, and I wasn't the neatest housekeeper.

When my labor with Ellie started, I demanded an epidural the minute I walked in the delivery room at Mount Auburn Hospital.

"You won't have enough time," the nurse said. "Second babies come fast."

"Let's just try," I encouraged her.

No one had met Ellie yet. She does things her way. I did get an epidural in time as Ellie was sunny-side up, which explained why the labor took so long and the pain was in my back. She eventually flipped and was born after midnight.

Spray lay on our gray rug. Even with ten puppies, she didn't cry out or make a mess. I bled, puked, pooped, and screamed when I pushed my babies out. Obviously, humans and dogs give birth differently. Dogs can't speak, so they don't count while bearing down. They can't push as long as humans do, and they don't sit up. When they deliver, a greenish bag of water often comes out before the puppy. While this is a bad sign in humans, it's perfectly normal in bitches.

As her puppies emerged, Spray didn't whimper or vomit on her doctor. She didn't walk around and howl, like the woman in the room next to me when I labored with Maggie.

I continued to sit next to Spray, leaning against the brown couch. I'm not a medical person. I faint when I see blood and get dizzy and lightheaded when people tell me their medical horror stories. But when my babies were born, I marveled at what the human body was capable of doing. Even though billions of women had done the same thing before me, I knew I was special and unique. Probably every woman has thought the same thing. Watching Spray give birth, I experienced similar disbelief that these little creatures had grown inside her for sixty-three days, and now she was giving them life.

After Laura wiped off the puppies, she held them out to Spray, who smelled and licked every one. Then Matt and Maggie placed them on a baby scale we had borrowed from Laura, where they wiggled around. Ellie wrote their weights next to a description of each of them on a large whiteboard. The biggest pup was eleven ounces, and the smallest was eight. We weighed them daily for a few weeks to make sure each was growing. After the weigh-in, we put them in a laundry basket, where they lay in a growing pile, one on top of the other, keeping each other company and warm.

We had a large box full of balls of colored yarn, similar to a box of crayons, also borrowed from Laura N., that we planned on using as collars for the little dogs. We identified the pups by the different color around each neck, but the natural coloring of our pups was unique. They were white, brown or black, with white, brown or black markings. It was easy to tell them apart. Because most PWDS are black, sometimes with little white accents, they can be hard to distinguish from one to another.

Maggie and Ellie thought the puppies were adorable. They cooed over the pups and wanted to hold them, but we left the litter alone with their mom. Slimy and wet, they didn't have much fur to speak of. When I posted photos on Facebook, a few people commented that the pups looked more like hamsters or guinea pigs than puppies. Their eyes were glued shut, and their ears were almost tacked back. Their eyes and ears opened a few weeks later. Their sense of smell, however, was intact from the moment they were born.

Spray, after her initial incident pushing away the first puppy, took to them immediately. Instantly, her maternal instincts kicked in.

Mine had been slower.

By the time Ellie was born, I understood, sort of, what a baby's needs were, but everything was new with Maggie. I didn't know how tired I could get. Unlike Spray, I didn't know how to nurse. Spray lay on the floor and let ten puppies climb all over her, searching for her nine teats. She never let on if nursing hurt. I had two nipples and one baby, and I struggled physically and emotionally.

After Maggie was born and the doctor announced she was a girl, the nurse cleaned her, wrapped her up and brought her to me. She lay on my chest, and I said, "It's nice to meet you."

Someone—the doctor or nurse—asked if we had a name.

Matt and I looked at each other. "What do you think?" I asked. "Elinor or Margaret?"

Who can say why one child looks like one name while another looks like another—but our first daughter looked like a Margaret. When Ellie was born, we chose between Caroline and Elinor, and we decided on Elinor.

After naming Maggie, the nurse asked if I wanted to breast-feed her. Until my children came along, I was modest, so I waited until I was in my private room, where I could decipher this nursing thing without a bunch of nurses and doctors watching. I assumed it would be a wonderful, natural, instinctual bonding experience with my baby. It wasn't. Every time Maggie latched on, my nipples felt like they were being pulled through an old-fashioned towel dryer.

The only things that helped were time and patience. Redheads, like me, I learned later have lower pain thresholds than blondes and brunettes. I was vindicated, not just about the breastfeeding, but for all my injuries and illnesses.

Once my nipples became tough as Tupperware, I kept at it until Maggie prompted me to wean her at eighteen months by biting me.

By the time Ellie came along, I was a nursing queen—nursing on planes, in restaurants, and at parks. My babies' needs trumped my modesty.

When I watched Spray nurse her puppies, I almost felt my milk let down, the way it had when Maggie and Ellie were hungry and cried years earlier.

By midmorning, nine of the puppies were born. Laura worked her magic and left us feeling more confident, and Maggie went to her chemistry exam. Ellie fell asleep on one of the sofas in the back room, and Matt and I sat staring at Spray and her tiny pups.

I wondered if Spray was as exhausted as she looked and if she thought about her puppies as she lay there suckling them.

After Maggie's birth on December 30, I had spent New Year's Eve in the hospital and watched the fireworks from my hospital window. When I fell asleep, I dreamed baby Maggie was cold, so I put her in an oven and turned it on. I woke in a total panic. Was this a sign? Was I doomed to fail as a mother?

Did dogs worry about their pups? About being a mother?

The baby blues hit when Maggie and I came home from the hospital. I lay in my bed, listening to my downstairs tenant coming in and out of his apartment at his leisure. I was now tethered to this other being. I would no longer be able to do anything without first considering Maggie. No matter what I was going to do, whether going to the grocery store for milk or returning to work, I reflected on how it would affect Maggie. A trip to the store involved dressing Maggie in warm clothes and carrying her with me. If I returned to work, I would need someone to watch Maggie. Every decision I made was influenced by this new being, and it continued like that for years.

Within a few weeks, however, I stopped missing my old life of easy come and go. I didn't miss the movies or the dinners out. Those were the easy sacrifices.

Maggie returned from her exam in time to catch the tenth and perhaps final puppy, another male, at 11:11. The lucky puppy. Ellie barely opened her eyes from the couch.

Soon after the tenth pup was born, Sandy and Jim arrived. They were eager to see the newborns and hoped to be there for some of the births. We still weren't sure whether an eleventh pup was tucked away somewhere, so Matt went to our local vet for a shot of oxytocin, known as a "clean out" injection, which he administered to Spray with Jim's help. This would encourage Spray's uterine horns to contract and, if there was another puppy in there, to push it out. We followed her outside when she did "her business" in case she gave birth out there. But there wasn't another puppy. Spray stopped at ten. Sandy and Jim reassured us that the puppies and Spray looked great.

We were in the clear. There had been no disasters. Now, we had to take care of puppies. Spray did most of the work in the beginning. After all the pups were born, we put them and Spray in the whelping box with a heating lamp and a space heater nearby. Not only was the room cold, but also, puppies can't regulate their internal temperatures for the first few weeks of life, so they need to stay warm—almost ninety degrees.

Even though Spray hadn't asked to be a mother, no one had to show her what to do. She counted her puppies by smelling them, and she knew when one wiggled away and nudged it back to the pack. She lay down with them to keep them warm, was available when they wanted to nurse, and even cleaned up after them, eating their little poops. We just did laundry. Lots of laundry.

Spray wouldn't leave her pups. Even when we knew she needed to go out again, no amount of cajoling could pull her away. Towards the end of the first day, we finally got her into the backyard, where she squatted, turned, and ran inside. There was no time to run and play. She had serious business to attend to.

Many breeders don't name their puppies, or they'll only call them by the colors around their necks. In theory, it's harder to get attached to nameless pups and easier to part with them. Laura, who went on to have more litters after her kids were out of college, named each of her Labrador litters by a theme—Laursans (named for Laura and Sandy) Labs named their litters *Harry Potter* characters, *Winnie the Pooh* names, herbs/spices, and a Christmas theme, among others.

Maggie and Ellie decided to name our litter Disney names, except for the one I named Map for the black markings on his white body.

Just as Matt and I named our daughters by what we saw in them at birth, the girls named the puppies. Laura asked them to give the second puppy a name with attitude, as she arrived with a strong personality. In birth order, we ended up with Mushu, Esmeralda, Map, Scar, Meeko, Pocahontas, Sarabi, Rafiki, Zazu, and Simba.

CHAPTER EIGHT

After the puppies were born, we hunkered down in the back room, our home within our home. Maggie and Ellie did their homework there, Matt watched TV, and I corrected papers. I couldn't have asked for a better life.

At first, we made sure someone was in the room with the puppies twenty-four seven. We sent Splash to stay with our dog walker, Scott, for two weeks, while Spray, the puppies, and the humans acclimated to their new world.

The puppies were completely dependent on Spray for their survival. By extension, they relied on us. Because Spray only had nine teats for ten pups, we needed to make sure the littlest dogs got turns suckling. Matt was the best at this, just as he had been an expert at swaddling our babies. He plucked the largest puppies like Map and Zazu off Spray and placed Mushu or Sarabi on so they got enough milk to grow. Then he weighed each pup to see what their growth was and marked it on the whiteboard.

The pups were like little bats zeroing in on Spray with radar. Their eyes were still closed so they used their sense of smell and heat sensors to find her and her milk. They wiggled their way around the whelping box like they were swimming. They couldn't stand and walk for a couple more weeks.

For the first week, we took turns sleeping in the back room.

Even though the whelping box had bumpers to prevent Spray from rolling over on the puppies, we wanted to make sure there weren't any accidents.

Ellie slept on the older, lumpier, oatmeal-colored sofa, while Matt pulled the cushions off the brown couch and put them on the floor next to the box, so he could reach in and move a pup if necessary. When it was my turn, I also slept on the oatmeal sofa, but I found it difficult to sleep through the night. It had nothing to do with my bedding or moving puppies. It was the chirping. The puppies chirped like seagulls throughout the night, like the birds that used to follow the ferry boat to the Vineyard hoping for handouts.

Once again, I was reminded of the sleepless nights with my own babies when they came home from the hospital and started adapting to the world. Their sleep habits were not in sync with mine. Babies and puppies aren't necessarily born with a proper sleep cycle built into their bodies. Eventually, sleep becomes more of a habit for the little ones, and the momma (human or dog) learns to sleep when her kids are asleep.

After the first week, we did leave the puppies, but not for more than two hours at a time. If we couldn't check on them, one of our dog walkers, Scott or Bray, did. But we really didn't have to worry. Spray was an excellent mother. She adjusted to her new role like she had planned for it. She didn't seem sad that she wasn't running around the backyard. But that would be anthropomorphizing Spray's behavior, which I was good at doing.

I didn't want to desert the puppies, but I did have to teach. I didn't want to miss one moment of growth, and I was guilt-ridden about leaving them when they might need me, which in hindsight was ridiculous—they needed Spray, not me, in the early days.

Matt stayed home from work when I went to Emerson, so

everyone really was well taken care of. I was envious—a natural state of mine—and I worried about them, much as I had with my own babies when I left them for the first time to return to work. I wanted to stay and protect them, hold and cuddle them, the way I had with my kids. To compensate for leaving the pups, I showed photos of them to my students and any colleagues I could corner into looking at them. I talked about them incessantly at school and at our neighborhood grocery store. I'm not sure what friends and colleagues thought. They were always polite and said, "How cute," or "Oh my God," or "So impressive." Were they really thinking: "She's nuts," or "That's a lot of puppies, good luck," or "Why?"

Spray lay in the whelping box in a crescent shape, and the puppies snuggled into her tummy, one on top of the other. If they weren't nursing, they lay on each other in twos and threes in different corners.

For six of the coldest weeks of winter, the back room—usually the frostiest in the house—was the warmest spot to be. We kept the door to the hall closed and the temperature cranked. We also opened the door to the basement so the heat from the furnace would rise. With the electric heater and lamp focused on the whelping box, the room stayed a toasty seventy-five degrees.

I fell in love with the puppies, harder and faster than predicted. Each was slowly developing its own personality, and I was growing attached to them as individuals and as a group. But, this was a business. We even named our kennel FayerWaves. "Fayer" was the first half of our street, Fayerweather, and "waves" was a nod to the water PWDs are so fond of. The puppies would leave after nine weeks. But, just as I fell for Maggie and Ellie as babies, knowing full well they would leave home one day, I was a goner for the pups. There was no way to protect myself—there was no wall high enough—to keep me from losing myself in my kids and puppies. Loss was coming.

I hadn't wanted either one of them, and yet there they were—and I was a better person for them. I learned more about myself and what I was capable of—helping to raise daughters, instilling in them the belief that they could do anything they set their minds to, and fighting for their rights with food allergies and sports.

Sometimes you don't know what you want until you're holding little hearts beating in your hands.

I obsessed over the puppies' health and growth. I took photos daily to chronicle their lives. I have hundreds upon hundreds of puppy photographs from one day to three months old on my computer and in two bound books. In the early stages of puppyhood, Spray did all the work, so it was easy and fun for us, and I wanted to share that joy and adventure with others. Even if people weren't dog people, most couldn't help being puppy people.

But as the puppies' growth and change slowed down, so did my postings. I figured not everyone in my virtual world was as fascinated by my pups as I was.

Much to my chagrin, Matt had been right about the puppies. It was a great adventure, one we all learned from.

When I came home after a long day of teaching, I'd find Maggie and/or Ellie lying on the back room couches with a puppy or two. Maggie no longer slunk off to her bedroom to chat online with friends. The four of us cooed and gawked, held and pet the puppies, together and alone. We all got a huge kick out of this, but we were also helping socialize the puppies by handling them as much as we were.

Newborn puppies shouldn't have visitors for their first two weeks of life. Not only do they need to bond with their mother, their siblings, and their human family, but they are also more susceptible to germs. The little dogs were changing daily, however, right in front of me, and when Susie, my dog-rescuing friend, said she wanted to see them, I couldn't resist showing off their rapid transformation.

Spray welcomed Laura when she came by to check on the puppies. She let Laura get close to the whelping box, stare into it and observe the puppies. Spray trusted her, as Laura had been such a big part of the birth. Jay, who spent a lot of time at our house, tiptoed into the back room to peek, and Spray hardly noticed. Neither of them tried to pick up a puppy. Only the immediate family was allowed that privilege.

Spray might not have asked to become a mom, but she became as protective of her children as I was of mine. When we moved the puppies to clean the whelping box, she followed each one out of the box. One day, instead of putting the puppies into a laundry basket while we changed the towels in the box, we put them, one by one, into Ellie's lap as she sat on the couch. Spray watched from the other end of the couch with a look of concern on her face, as if she was thinking, "Don't mess with those pups…You do know they're mine."

But on the day Susie came to visit, Spray's reaction went way beyond concern. As Susie approached the threshold to the back room, Spray leapt from the whelping box and ran to the doorway, baring her teeth and growling in a manner I'd never witnessed.

She had a message to deliver, and she did so loud and clear. Susie backed down the hallway and didn't come in for another week. We learned our lesson. Spray wasn't looking at a calendar, but instinctively she knew the puppies weren't ready for guests.

Just as my role evolved as my kids grew up, Spray's would too. When Maggie and Ellie were young, my responsibilities were easier to define. I fed them, played with them, bathed them, read to them, walked them to school and back, but as they became teenagers, my role underwent a seismic shift. Collecting the chestnuts that fell from the big tree in our neighborhood wasn't as exciting for them as it had been when they were little and we did it together every fall. I could no longer sing my lyrics to the Manfred Mann song. "There they were just a-walking down the street, singing do wah diddy diddy dum diddy o." As they matured, their lives would take them further away from me. I had known that since the moment each of them was born. With that first breath they took out of the womb, they were starting to separate from me.

I also didn't know in the early days of parenting that I would change. I knew what kind of mother I was going to be—no pacifiers, no children in our bed, only six months of nursing. I was going to maintain some of my independence.

That didn't work. You guessed it—I followed my daughters' leads. Maggie weaned herself at eighteen months, but she fell in love with pacifiers. She slept on her back in her crib, surrounded by as many as we could throw in, so she could reach out and grab one. Occasionally, she slept with us. Ellie, however, was claustrophobic, and no amount of Ferber (letting her cry it out) convinced her that the crib was a good place. So, the family bed arrived at our house.

I didn't want to be judged by my family or friends, so I didn't always share my parenting decisions. Mothers, especially, are quick to judge one another, when really, they should be supporting each other regardless of their parenting styles.

We wanted well-adapted puppies. Shy or reserved pups could be harder to manage, like Splash. Well socialized pups, like Spray, get along with everyone and aren't afraid of school buses and motorcycles.

The puppies quickly got used to being held incessantly. It was virtually impossible to be in the back room and not pick up a puppy from the whelping box. When Maggie or Ellie held them, the puppies sucked on their noses and ears. They didn't bark or growl yet; rather, they continued chirping like squeaky toys. Their breath smelled like a nice skunk smell, if there is such a thing. When the little dogs weren't sleeping on top of one another, in what was truly a puppy pile, they wiggled and squirmed their way around the whelping box, like live versions of Maggie's baby toy, Wiggle Worm.

Puppies, with their round tummies and nuzzling noses, make everything right in the world, if just for a moment.

Ellie said it best: "Whenever I'm sad, I just pick up a puppy."

Holding a puppy in my hands, letting one lie on my chest or watching them play together was peaceful. The world couldn't be a bad place if it had room for puppies.

My puppies encouraged me to live in the moment, and forget about the articles I had to write, the papers I had to correct, my daughters' homework, and college applications. For just that moment, the world shrank to just me and a puppy or two. They made me feel needed and, just like babies, they represented a promise about the future. Otherwise known as *puppy meditation.*

When new parents ask me for advice, I say to do what's best for their children. They'll know. I tell them not to listen to those who have differing opinions and to ignore the unsolicited advice people want to offer. But be prepared, I say, your life is about to change in ways you never thought possible. The whole focus and purpose of your life shifts after you have a baby.

Did dogs obsess about their changing lives the way I fixated about mine?

When the puppies were two weeks old and a bit more independent, and Spray separated from them a bit, we welcomed visitors, including Susie, into our home. We also invited Splash home after his two-week stay with Scott. Ironically, as the scary dog in the house, he was afraid of the puppies. He stayed as far away as possible, once getting backed into a corner by the puppies.

Guests arrived in droves. We couldn't have asked for a better mix to help us socialize the pups. People of all ages and races trooped through our doors. Neighbors and parents from school stopped by. Family, colleagues, some of my students, my kids' friends and some friends I hadn't seen in a long time dropped by, along with prospective buyers. Our home was busy and even more chaotic than usual.

I loved it.

I finally had a legitimate reason for a messy *and* smelly house. For once, I wasn't conflicted between wanting a neat house like I had grown up with—where my mother insisted we plump the sofa pillows after we sat on them—and wanting the clutter of lacrosse sticks on the front porch and boots and backpacks in the front hall, that showed a family in action. I didn't have time to freak out about what people thought of our entryway or whether the kids picked up their books in the living room. I didn't care, and no one else seemed to, either. We were in the midst of life, and it was hectic.

I also didn't worry about entertaining. Neither my friends nor my daughters' friends cared if they were offered coffee, tea, a brownie or cookie, all of which were usually available in our home. They came for the puppies, to see them romp with each other or just to watch them curl up on top of each other. One of Ellie's friends, Maddy, sat on the couch with Pocahontas on her lap and said, "Now I see why you talk about the puppies all the time."

Some guests simply wanted to watch Spray's whole family play.

Some fell in love with a specific puppy and focused their attention on that pup. Either way, visitors did us an enormous favor by helping us with the necessary and important job of socializing the puppies. The more callers, the more socializing. We wanted well socialized pups, not fearful, shy, and unfriendly ones. You want puppies to be calm and unafraid of noise.

We were determined to deliver friendly little dogs to their new owners. They were going to be well-grounded pups.

While the puppies still played and slept together most of the time, Matt started to separate them occasionally so they could begin to learn what it was like to be on their own. He took one or two upstairs to our main living space.

But before all those changes, the puppies explored the second floor. They cruised around, investigating the couch upstairs and the rug on the floor, as well as scooting under the dining room chairs.

Matt also took them one at a time for car rides, their first of many. He even took Map to church one day, as he slid around on the passenger seat.

Matt was the puppies' personal tour guide of Cambridge and life inside a car. "Now, this is a car seat you'll grow into," he might have said. "The window is for looking out of. That's Harvard Square, where I took Morgie on our first date. And that's the river, and this is a bridge we're going over."

The puppies' eyes and ears opened, and they went from chewing on each other and growling at one another into a more boisterous stage. We packed up the whelping box after four weeks and bought a plastic indoor play pen. They crawled around and wrestled with toys and humans alike, whether in the playpen or on the carpet in the back room.

They could finally go outside, although it took them a while to learn to go down the porch steps. We carried them down two at a time. But before we could get any more down, the first two ran back up, so we carried them back down. It was a game. We watched them run through leaf piles, play tug of war and gnaw on twigs in the yard. Map often stood on a heap of leaves like he was king of the hill.

Before they learned the art of going down stairs, we staged them on the back porch at the top of the stairs, calling out to them to *sit* and *stay*, which they didn't understand. Matt held Spray by her collar at the bottom of the stairs. I had a camera. I clicked photo after photo until I got one of all ten sitting in a row. I won a prize for it in the Martha's Vineyard Ag Fair, and it hangs in our house as well as many of the puppies' forever homes. I gave a framed copy to Maggie and Ellie when they left for college—a reminder of our great family adventure.

My father, a retired architect/developer, who lived in England, was also an artist. Several of his landscapes hang on our walls. Most of them reflect a place he has lived: the Berkshires, Portugal, and the English countryside. The surprise he created for us was a painting based on the iconic puppy photograph. It's one of the first things you see coming into our home.

Spray's interaction with her puppies was instinctual. She didn't overthink what she was doing, the way mothers can. If a puppy got out of line by being too rambunctious with a sibling, she snarled and bopped it with her paw. She didn't worry about what might happen later that afternoon, let alone for the rest of her life, like I might have done.

Puppies and dogs eat, sleep, play, pee and poop, and then repeat. They react to the moment they're in. They don't look ahead; they don't look back. Spray nursed her pups, guarded them, and slept when she could. She protected her pups, but I don't know if she loved her progeny the way I loved my children. She wasn't invested in their futures or health the way I was. I worried about Maggie's allergies, making friends, and her future at college. How would we redefine ourselves as a family after she left? Animals are created to let their offspring go, while humans are connected for life. I was apprehensive about my future and nostalgic about what had already passed.

When I nursed my daughters, I reveled in the time I had alone with them, their bodies curving into mine, their tiny hands pawing at my breasts and their mouths pulling at my nipples for the warm milk. When Maggie and Ellie stopped, they were moving on to a different phase of their lives, one in which I was less essential. My role changed—subtly at first, but change was coming. The girls were leading me, and I had to keep up, to adapt. This pattern of leading and following would continue for the rest my life.

If I could handle the sadness at weaning my children, maybe I wouldn't be so sad when they went to kindergarten, sleep-away camp, and college or when they got married.

I was wrong.

Before Spray had the puppies, she leapt about, chased Splash and danced in circles, but all that stopped when she became a mother. She didn't run anymore. Her rollicking gait slowed. She was sedate and kept a watchful eye on the pups. Had we changed her forever? Was it good? Had we made a mistake? I also transformed when I had kids, but at the core, I was probably more me than ever. I learned to trust my instincts when it came to my children and their needs. My social life was smaller, but I didn't miss it as I nestled into my life at home.

Change can be scary, but it's not always bad. Sometimes, it's exciting.

Some breeders separate the dam and her pups during the weaning stage, keeping them apart for three days while the pups are introduced to goat's milk or formula.

I couldn't do that. Just like I couldn't stand listening to Ellie cry when we tried to get her to sleep in a crib. The thought of intentionally splitting the puppies from Spray, even if it made weaning easier, crushed my heart. I didn't want to hear Spray scratching at the door to come in, and I didn't want to hear the pups bleating for their mom. Matt and I believed in letting nature take its course, so we let Spray wean her pups her way, the way I had with my daughters.

When Spray entered the back room, her teats swinging below her, the pups ran to her and tried to grab hold, their heads tilted back with open mouths, but Spray kept walking as the pups let go and fell to the floor. Often, she ran through the room and leapt up on the sofa, to sit where her babes couldn't reach her. Even when she willingly lay down to nurse the little dogs, she stood when she was done, and the pups dangled and plopped to the floor. Her message was clear: *I'm closing up shop. Get used to it. Get with the program*—one of my mother's favorite expressions.

Spray inspired me. Somehow, she knew not only when to look after her pups but also when to take her own needs and wants into account. Even if I hadn't wanted to nurse anymore, I'm not sure I had the guts to shut the dairy bar. I put my kids' needs and desires, whether physical or emotional, before my own. Only when Maggie went to college did I really start paying attention to what I wanted to do with my life.

While Spray decreased her nursing, we introduced the pups to food. We started with Gerber's Rice Cereal combined with a formula we made from condensed milk and corn syrup. Matt used the immersion blender—which I had given him to make soup—to mix it. The result was sticky and messy. The toothless puppies dove into it, getting it on their backs and heads, and then licked it off each other.

Initially, all ten puppies fit around the "flying saucer" feeding dish we had borrowed from Sandy and Jim. It was a round dish with a large hump in the middle, which created a trough for the pups' food. But as they grew bigger, we divided them into two eating groups of five each.

After a week of baby cereal, they graduated to kibble mush—puppy chow mashed up with more of the homemade formula. Matt smashed it together so it was easier for them to lap up and digest. The puppies' teeth started to come in at about five weeks when they learned to chew their food, though they had not yet mastered the art of keeping it in the dish. They excelled at dropping food on one another, their toys, and stuffed animals.

With real food came real poop with real smell. The house started to assume the aroma of a kennel. Spray resigned from her job of keeping things clean. It was our turn.

The little dogs also started to play together more—pawing, wrestling, and chewing one another. As the weather warmed, we let them out onto the back porch more, where they learned to pee, poop, and skid around.

While Spray was slowly letting go of her pups and letting visitors in to see them, she was still protective. If her old buddy Splash came into the room on his way to the back door, she placed herself between him and the puppies.

Splash, however, didn't need anyone to protect the puppies from him. He was terrified of them, as with many moving objects. If they were loose in the room, they ran up to him en masse when he entered, pinning him in a corner where he sat and barked at them, waiting to be rescued.

Just as I had evolved after Maggie and Ellie were born, Spray changed too. She was still sweet, slept with Matt and ran away when he sneezed, but the protective side she developed as a mom remained. I left her in my car one day with the windows partly down in a parking lot on the Vineyard. From the store's front counter, I heard her barking sharply at someone putting their hand inside the window to pet her. She may have tried to bite the hand. As much as she shouldn't, I didn't blame her. Who puts their hand inside a stranger's car?

Spray protected her puppies, just as I advocated for Maggie and Ellie in ways I never imagined possible before I had kids. While I'm not great at speaking up for myself, I'm ferocious when it comes to my children.

Maggie was part of the first wave of kids who had life-threatening allergies to peanuts and tree nuts. When Maggie was three, Matt and I began looking for preschools.

"How do you take care of the kids who have allergies during snack?" I asked at one.

"We try to encourage the children to look out for themselves," came the answer. We opted out of that school. She ended up at a small cooperative preschool where parents were involved on a daily basis.

When Maggie was ready for kindergarten, we investigated our options. The large lunchrooms in the public schools frightened me because Maggie would have so little control over who sat next to her and what they brought for lunch. After much discussion, we applied to a few independent schools, and Maggie ended up at the one I had graduated from years earlier and Matt had attended when he was young.

The world is different since Maggie was in kindergarten, with more awareness around food allergies and their dangers. Most children develop food allergies in the first two years of life. That was true for Maggie, but not for either Matt or Ellie, who were older. Between the time Maggie was diagnosed at the end of 1992, up until 2007, the prevalence of reported food allergies increased 18 percent among children under age 18 years.

Some kids have died. Each time I read about a death, my heart skipped a beat and my stomach sank. Still does.

Not only did I worry about protecting both Matt and Maggie, but Ellie also developed allergies to many foods, especially tomatoes, in high school. Keeping them safe became my life's mission.

One evening, when I was helping feed the cast and crew of a play Ellie was in, her face broke out in light pink hives, almost like blush. I had never seen this before, and because Maggie was away, I didn't have an EpiPen with me. As Ellie's breathing became more labored and she was dizzy, another student gave me his Epi, and without thinking much about it, I jabbed it into Ellie's thigh and counted to ten. The first responders arrived and took her to a hospital. That was the first of many.

Many schools are nut-free now, but in the mid-1990s, this was not yet the case. Not only did the school say it would work with us to make Maggie safe, but also, Matt and I liked its academic mission. The school was traditional in its approach to education but became more innovative the longer we were there. It was the perfect fit for Maggie, but when Ellie moved from grade to grade, we realized it wasn't the right match for everyone, even siblings. Safeguarding Maggie and educating those around her in the lower, middle, and upper schools took a lot of time and energy. Each time I advocated for her, I also let go of her a little more. The lower school created safe classrooms for Maggie; they were nut-free. This didn't sit well with some families, who were convinced their children only ate peanut butter. As someone who grew up on peanut butter, I understand the attachment, but when a child's life is in the balance, even I, who ate not much else, chucked it.

When Maggie started middle school (grades seven through eight), I asked for a nut-free zone in the "great room" where the students brought and ate their lunches. I wasn't making much headway, until I presented the middle school director with an obituary of a young woman who had died from anaphylaxis. Suddenly, there was a nut-free table. In high school, students kept their food on trays, away from Maggie. The older she got, the more responsible she became for herself and the environments in which she was eating.

I crossed my fingers as her world grew larger and she stepped further away from me. Obsessing about Matt and Maggie was consuming. Hearing a horrible story made me that much more crazed. Nobody knows what's going to get them in the end—it could be a bus or cancer—but knowing that something like a nut, apple, or tomato could potentially kill someone I love is terrifying. The fear hovered above my head like a whirring helicopter.

Ellie had her own battles with OCD and ADHD. She worked hard to hold it together at school, falling apart when she got home.

Matt and I talked with her teachers about how to use her learning style to assist her.

"Ellie is a literal person," I explained. "I told her to take a shower one day, and when she came downstairs, I asked if she had washed her hair. 'No,' she said. 'You didn't tell me to.'"

She avoided the reading corner in fifth grade not because she was defiant, as her teacher told us, but because she was a slow processor and was anxious about her reading ability compared to her classmates, many of whom were reading two grade levels ahead.

Ellie wasn't happy. The kids in her class weren't particularly nice to her, some called her names, and the teachers didn't understand her learning style. We were all frustrated. She was lucky that she got one teacher for two years—third and fourth grade—who understood Ellie, and encouraged us to move her from this high-powered traditional school.

In fifth grade, Ellie applied to and was accepted at another school that focused more on the whole student and prided itself on teaching a myriad learning styles, especially those children with ADHD.

Within two weeks of Ellie's sixth grade year, she got in my car after school one day and said, "I'm smart, Mummy. I'm smart."

CHAPTER NINE

I wondered if our puppies were pooped from growing so fast. If a one-year-old puppy is equal to a seven-year-old human, just imagine their first year of life.

That's a lot of developing in a short span of time. My daughters didn't stand up and begin walking until nearly a year old, but in a matter of weeks, the pups stopped swimming across the whelping box. They stood on wobbly legs and exhibited what we dubbed "the dinosaur walk" as they lurched forward and lunged sideways.

The pups would continue to mature at their forever homes. They would rush through toddlerhood and childhood and enter adolescence all within the first year of life. Not only would they keep transforming, but also, the owners would have to keep up with them. It could be challenging at times; chewing and house-training were going to give the new owners something to work on.

Puppy school and obedience training are essential. Puppies, like children, have a hard time regulating themselves and will play or run even when they're tired and should rest. Therefore, it's up to parents—or in this case, humans—to make sure the pups had time to be quiet, in a pen or crate.

But, we still had them for a few more weeks before their forever homes started loving and caring for them. The pups turned into fluff balls that rolled around on the gray carpet together and then slept on top of each other. We spent hours sitting on one of our couches, watching them. Of course, holding them was also delicious.

The little dogs completely disrupted our family life. Our routines—morning and evening in particular—were shot. Friends visited all day long, but the puppies bonded the four of us together in our mission to care for them and raise them to be the best dogs. We were a team, just as Matt and I were a team raising Maggie and Ellie.

We lived by the puppies' schedule, not the one we were used to. We woke earlier than usual to feed them their mushy food and take them outside. We tried to encourage housebreaking before the pups moved out. We were somewhat successful, but as I heard once, "Your dog is either housebroken or not. It can't be 'sort of' housebroken."

We ate our own breakfast after we took care of the puppies. The girls ate Cheerios, Matt liked Kashi, and I went for Frosted Flakes or Rice Krispies. Ellie and I were in a carpool to her school, and Maggie walked or Matt gave her a ride to hers. In a few weeks, Maggie would be done with classes. After March vacation, she moved onto her Senior Project for the last part of her senior year, which consisted of directing the senior play, reading in a mystery book club, and singing with the Senior Voices, part of Chorale.

Puppies, like babies, represent hope and the promise of better opportunities. Our babies, Maggie and Ellie, provided Matt and me with the prospect of stepping away from some of our past, where we didn't always feel we were the first thought on our parents' minds. Our kids, we decided, would be our priority. We rarely left them for our own time together, but we focused on what we thought was right for them. As all parents find out, we aren't perfect, and even if you try not to make mistakes, you do—just different ones from the ones your parents made.

By the time I was fourteen, I had lived in eight houses, in four cities in two countries. I discovered much later that relocating with Matt was much more fun than my memories of relocating when I was a child. Feeling safe, loved, and part of the decision-making had a lot to do with that.

But I didn't know that for years, and Matt and I hunkered down in Cambridge, raising our kids in the same house they came home to from the hospital. Thirty years later, we are still there (with a one-year hiatus).

When my mother and her kids returned from London in 1968, we went straight to the Vineyard and Grandma. I never saw the inside of our home in New York again, though I visited my father at various apartments in the city monthly. At the end of the summer, my mother moved the three kids, once again, this time to Cambridge. I started at another new school, and we moved into our first rental on Farrar Street. A year later, we moved to Lakeview Avenue. When I was thirteen, my mother remarried, and we moved into a new home, where my mom and Dads stayed for a quarter-century.

But I don't remember anyone saying they were sorry for how the divorce, moves, and remarriages affected me. I didn't hear any apologies for the lack of trust I developed and the loneliness that enveloped me. They were too busy taking care of themselves, recreating lives from the burnt embers left around the fires they created.

In high school, I had hung out on my friend Philip's third floor. There, I trusted my friends as we passed lighted joints around the room, where we sat on cushions watching fish swim in the vast aquarium or the Celtics when their games were on TV.

My mother, along with two stepmothers, are gone. But my father and stepfather have stayed loyal, and as our relationships grew stronger, they stood by and watched me learn to trust myself as I married Matt and grew a family I hadn't planned on having.

I wanted my children to have the stability I had lacked—a neighborhood and a home. A side benefit was, I thrived as well. I also fit into this world. I was part of the customers with charge accounts at the grocery store around the corner from our house. Shopping there was more than picking up pasta and milk. The store provided the space and opportunity for neighbors and friends, and in my case family, to bump into each other and chat about their lives.

Years later, I realized I had recreated my New York neighborhood—living in a vertical home, around the corner from a retail center and across the street from two girls Maggie and Ellie's age, who are still best friends.

When my mother died, I hid in Fresh Pond Market beside the paper towels, afraid of crying if anyone said hi or asked how I was. I bumped into someone I knew there all the time. Often my cousin, Betsy, who lived a few blocks away, and I shopped at the same time. When that happened, we holed up in a corner to talk about our parents or kids.

Mark and Crosby, the owners and brothers, welcomed every visitor into their store like we were their best friends. They knew so many family stories. The day they closed the store in September of 2019, after almost one hundred years in their family, the street and sidewalk were packed with well-wishers who were sad the store was closing, but happy for them. Little did we know the pandemic was lurking—they timed closing up perfectly.

The stores on the street were supporting characters in my daughters' lives. All the storekeepers knew them; they'd watched my girls grow up and knew when they performed plays or had a voice concert. Maggie and Ellie worked their first jobs around the corner. The older I got, and the more Maggie and Ellie were living their lives—with boyfriends and school—I loved checking in with the storekeepers, like Judy, Melissa, or Billy from the dress shop J. Miles (where three generations of women in my family have shopped); or Sarah from our favorite eatery, Full Moon, who gave Matt real maple syrup for his pancakes, and Maggie a job.

As the weather warmed up in March, I sat outside more often. The puppies chased each other; Map headed to his leaf pile and Mushu and Simba tumbled, while Sarabi and Esmeralda played tug of war with a stick. The puppies frolicked, running in circles around each other, but they also paired off and cavorted with their favorite littermates.

When the puppies were six weeks old, we packed all ten into two plastic laundry baskets to take them to the vet for their first round of shots and microchipping. Dr. Emara, who I had started visiting when I was single with a cat, had seen me through my adult stages of getting married, having kids, adding one dog to our family and then a second. Now he was part of our puppy adventure. He retired by the time we added Mayzie and Lily.

Dr. Emara closed his office during our visit. The puppies had full run of the place. They ran in and out of examining rooms, skidding down the linoleum hallway in the waiting area while the vet techs chased them and took pictures. Our gentle, kind, and reserved vet smiled and laughed while the multicolored pups slid and flailed around his space.

I lugged puppies in the laundry baskets to visit Maggie and Ellie at school. We called it *Puppy Therapy*. When the pups were young and small, they all fit in one basket. But as they got older and bigger, we couldn't squeeze as many into the baskets, and it was taxing trying to keep them in place as they tried to climb out.

Parents and students I didn't know stopped me in hallways to ask about the puppies, as well as to pet and coo over them.

At Maggie's school, football jocks who had never spoken to her lay down on the floor and let the little dogs crawl over them. Rafiki went into the head of the upper school's office and mistook it for the outdoors. Luckily, Mr. Knapp had a good sense of humor. When he retired at the end of the year, I sent him a photo of Maggie and Rafiki.

I hauled another load of puppies to Ellie's school, and her math teacher delayed the start of class as the puppies staggered around the classroom floor we covered with newspaper. Word traveled fast that puppies were on campus, and an ongoing line of teachers and students snaked its way in and out of the classroom to see and play with them.

The puppies and I visited Matt at Massport. His colleagues stuck their heads out their office doors and then stepped completely into the hall to watch the pups run up and down the corridor. Everyone grinned to see the pups' adventures.

No matter where we went, we carried a roll of paper towels and a spray bottle just in case.

When I was with our dogs on the Vineyard or out for a walk on the two-mile loop around Fresh Pond in Cambridge, they enabled me to live in the moment. The dogs wanted sticks thrown for them. They wanted to dive into the waves. Alone with them, I forgot about the papers sitting on my desk at home or my children's needs.

For those few moments, the world was just my dogs and me. I stopped worrying about Maggie and college or about how I fit in with my friends or whether I did a good job in the classroom. The puppies and dogs kept my insecurities tamped down.

Dogs don't have the verbal capacity to tell you what's going on, but they do have emotions, and you can see what they're feeling if you look at their faces closely. If we paid enough attention, we could learn something from them. As humans, we tend to look ahead and back. Why not savor this moment, instead?

Jim and Sandy Nightingale warned us that the hardest part of breeding had nothing to do with caring for the puppies. It was managing the human element—the people interested in buying them.

They were right.

When the pups were four weeks old, the Nightingales visited to see how Cocoa's grandchildren were developing. They sat on our brown couch, amidst the smell and chaos of the back room.

"Pay attention to your gut," Jim said. "You're responsible for these pups. You're acting on Spray's behalf."

I finally understood why the breeders from whom we purchased our two dogs interrogated us like we were spies. They wanted to make sure they were handing their pups over to a responsible family who would love them and incorporate them into their lives.

Jim was right. I was surprised at how protective I was of the pups. They were my responsibility. We made sure they all went to loving and welcoming homes. Easy.

Some buyers only care about what a prospective puppy looks like—how cute they are and what color they are. This is a mistake. Buyers should pay more attention to the puppy's personality and how it will fit in with their home life. An outgoing pup might work well in a home with kids. A quieter dog might be better for a single, older person.

Some breeders decide who will get what dog, without asking for the buyer's opinion. Breeders know their puppies and their temperaments and what kind of home they fit best.

We knew one of our three females was going home with Mervan and Lucy. We just didn't know which one. They wanted one of the brown girls, and so did we, but I couldn't decide whether Esmeralda or Sarabi fit in our family better. I loved both, but choosing one meant actively *not* choosing the other. I am terrible at making decisions. Choices and decisions involve loss, and I don't do loss well, but I doubt the puppies had any idea of my agony.

Meanwhile, Mervan visited frequently, eager to find out which pup would be his.

Most of the prospective buyers came to us through word of mouth. We eliminated many through preliminary phone interviews, after which we met and interviewed the others. I respected those who took themselves out of the buying process when they realized the breed wasn't right for them, either because the dogs weren't as hypoallergenic as they hoped, were too rambunctious for a family with young kids, or needed too much exercise and attention.

We never came out and said "no" to anyone, but we counseled buyers to consider the commitment they were making to the dog and the breed. We reminded them of PWDs' high energy, need for incessant exercise and constant companionship, as well as their insatiable appetite for eyeglasses, tables, and shoes. We were ready to tell one family whose son couldn't wait to shoot Nerf balls at his new dog that they rethink the breed, but luckily, they went another direction without our counsel.

Matt and I never intended to piss anyone off, but our first responsibility was to the pups and Spray. We wanted to err on the side of caution. We'd rather wait longer to get the right person than move fast to get them out of our house. We wanted to sleep well at night, knowing we had done our best. Plus, I was in no hurry to see them go.

Once the families and forever homes had been determined, we needed to select the right pup for each home. The early buyers told us their first three choices, and then we assessed which one was be best suited to them and their lifestyles.

Initially, everyone wanted the one female available, assuming she was the quietest of the bunch, but I was pleasantly surprised to discover most of the males had inherited Spray's demeanor and were calmer than the typical male PWD. As I meet more and more Portuguese water dogs, I see just how unusual Splash was and that I shouldn't use him as a measuring stick for male PWDs.

Matt, Maggie, Ellie, and I understood the individual personalities of the puppies. We knew which ones were quiet and sedate and which were rambunctious. We wanted to make sure we matched puppy temperaments to prospective homes.

To ensure we were making the right calls, we turned once more to Laura N., who ran the puppies through a series of tests to determine their temperaments. We didn't know how to do this, and it was better if a stranger did the testing to accurately gauge the pups' responses. The puppies knew us too well.

Laura visited on a day when two families stopped by to find out which pup would be theirs. They had come before and narrowed their choices, but now the pups were six weeks old, and it was time to match the puppies with their new homes. While we sat in the living room chatting and the remaining little dogs crawled around the rug, Laura took each puppy into a room behind a closed door so she could evaluate them away from the pack mentality.

First, she hit the floor to gauge the pups' reactions. Did they startle? Were they scared, hostile, or inquisitive? Or did they ignore her?

After the startle test, she called them with a happy voice to test their engagement. This determined who immediately engaged with her and came at her call, who was timid, who paused but eventually came, and again, who had no interest at all.

For the last test, she turned the puppies over on their backs and gently held them, while reassuring them. This showed her who was timid, who submitted, who was anxious but could be calmed, and who just plain didn't like it.

"As you can see, it really gives you a sense of a calm dog, an inquisitive dog, the timid dog who probably needs no kids, and an alpha which you can train and can be great if you are an alpha," she said.

Her findings corroborated ours. We knew Simba, Zazu, and Meeko were the calmest, while Map, Ezzie, and Mushu were at the other end of the hyper spectrum. Simba went to the South End, and Mushu went to Newton.

Just as I wanted Maggie to end up at the college that fit her the best, I wanted the puppies to fit seamlessly into their new homes. The wrong fit for a puppy or Maggie could be problematic. If the puppy didn't work out, the owner was required to return it to us, and I didn't want any more dogs. Three was enough. If Maggie wasn't happy at the college she selected, the consequences could be complicated. Fixable, but complicated.

When it was time to choose the puppy to stay with us, the decision was made easier by the pup, herself. In the end, Esmeralda chose me. Every time I came into the back room, she trotted over, rubbed against my legs, and looked up at me, as if she were reminding me to pick her up and hold her.

Sarabi, her look-alike, didn't seem interested in me, although when I visited her later at Mervan and Lucy's, she turned in circles and jumped at me in recognition and ecstasy. I was a rock star. Mervan and Lucy have had two babies since Sparky's arrival—as they renamed her—and they became best friends. Sparky popped up on Facebook periodically, running on the grounds of the boarding school where Mervan now works and lives. I always commented: "SPARKY"!

We tried to come up with a water name for Esmeralda, to complement Splash and Spray, but we couldn't come to a consensus on Sprite or Spout. She already knew her own spunky Disney name—Ezzie for Esmeralda—so we kept it.

The puppies began leaving months before Maggie went to college, but I found it impossible not to project ahead. I imagined the pit in my stomach I felt about the dogs leaving would be magnified when it was Maggie's turn to walk out the door and close it behind her.

The new owners were excited to be adding onto their families, bringing new joy into their lives. Although we found loving homes for the puppies, I started to break inside when I handed them over. I became tied to them. Now I had to rip those ties. They would no longer be my puppies; they were going to their forever homes, much like when Maggie got married years later. She would always be my daughter, but she was a wife now with her own family. While the pups started with us, and some did remember us for years, they were with their families now. As it should be.

Watching how happy the new families were made me feel better. We gifted these families love in the form of a puppy.

I didn't have to wait until Maggie got married to feel her loss. While she was still connected to me through our history, love, phones, and computers when she left for school, she was also stepping into her own separate life, also as she should. But I missed the everyday with her. She would never live at home again. Her room remained her room for years, there for her to visit, until we moved away temporarily, and I cleaned it out for renters. Later, it became my sewing room, and the dining room returned to its traditional use.

Before the new dog owners arrived at our house, we all took turns holding the puppy who was moving on to their forever home. We cuddled with them and took pictures. We all lunged for the pup, each wanting a chance to say goodbye.

Each time a pup left, Matt distracted Spray with a piece of chicken left over from one of my roast chicken meals. After I said goodbye and the door shut behind the new larger families, Spray returned. She didn't look for the missing pup, didn't cry, or count the remaining pups. She resumed her life as though nothing of consequence had happened.

Chicken was not going to do it for me when Maggie left. I was going to definitely notice her absence.

I don't like saying goodbye. But I hoped saying goodbye to the puppies was good practice and I'd be okay when Maggie left. But as much as I loved them and cried when they left, they were puppies. Maggie was my daughter.

It was easy to love all the puppies, individually and as a pack, but we also created some special bonds. Maggie loved Rafiki; Matt had a thing for Mushu, the pup he saved at birth; Ellie loved them all but thought Sarabi was pretty; and I fell for crazy, hard-to-control Map, the son I never had, as well as Ezzie, who slept with me.

After several weeks, a few puppies—including Map, Rafiki, Pocahontas and Mushu—still didn't have permanent homes, although lots of people visited. As time went on, we wondered if we were being too particular. We could easily have sold three times as many puppies if we hadn't been so careful with our decision-making. But ultimately, every pup ended up in the perfect forever home.

One of the last to go was Pocahontas, the third girl. The family was renaming her Molly, my mother's name. Maggie came home from school for lunch that day because she knew I might struggle saying goodbye.

I looked at Maggie and then away. I didn't want to cry. I waved my hands in front of my eyes to stop my whimpering. My mother would have thought I'd lost my mind breeding Spray. I missed her, especially because she was an active and involved grandmother who had helped me when the kids were little. But I didn't worry about her opinions anymore. I was a little freer to be me and to spend time with my husband. Perhaps we could start going to the theater or out to dinner, just the two of us.

With the departure of each dog, the house got quieter and quieter.

Sandy and Jim told us we would be glad to see the last puppy leave after spending weeks cleaning up after them, but I wasn't relieved, even though Ezzie joined our family. I was empty and lonely, the way I expected I'd feel when Maggie left, taking her sparkling brown eyes, dark brown hair, her calm, and her smile with her.

Later in April, after most of the puppies had found new families and homes and left our house, Maggie and I returned to Vassar for a revisit day. She had been accepted at this point and needed to decide where she wanted to enroll for the fall. The field hockey coach wanted her as a goalie, and Matt and I thought the school was a good fit, and not because Matt and I were alums. The school had strong drama and film departments, areas of interest to Maggie. It was close to New York, but not in the city, and it was out of our state, something she insisted upon. Maggie, however, still said it felt more like a boarding school, and she didn't see anyone with whom she thought she could be friends. How she could determine this by looking at the students walking by was lost on me. She was angry, and I was exasperated.

As we sat in the Retreat, the school's coffee shop, later that day, I texted Matt: *You would be so frustrated with her right now.*

Maggie looked up from her phone and said, "Would I?" I had sent the message to her.

We moved from the Retreat back to our car, where we sat and discussed her options, staring through the front window.

"You don't have to go here," I said. "Take a gap year."

"I don't know. There's no one here that looks like me."

"Transfer. Try one of the other schools, and if you don't like it, transfer."

Maggie remained unmoved and unconvinced.

She was not a natural extrovert. Maggie had not been a party girl in high school. Asked to describe herself, she probably would say she was a geek. She stayed home on the weekends and watched movies either by herself or with a small group of other non-partier friends. *Harry Potter* was her love.

When I suggested she go to a party that evening, she said, "No."

"You don't even have to drink at it," I said. "Get a cup, fill it with soda or water, and hang onto it so it looks like you're drinking, but don't take a drink from anyone else."

I couldn't believe I was pushing her to go to a party; what role reversal.

My persuasion worked. Maggie went to two parties with people she had met when she slept over with the field hockey team several months previously.

At one, the Backstreet Boys song "Shape of My Heart" came on, and the partiers shouted the lyrics. Finally, Maggie told me later, she had found her peeps and she could see herself at Vassar. I wanted to send a card to the Backstreet Boys to thank them.

By the next morning, she was all about Vassar. Matt arrived midmorning as reinforcement to help convince Maggie that this was the school for her, but it wasn't necessary. Maggie had made up her mind. We met the field hockey coach and team, and she learned about the drama and film departments. At the end of the day, we went to the college store to buy Vassar paraphernalia, including stickers for our cars.

Years later, Maggie can hardly remember where else she applied. Vassar and she fit together, just like the pups in the right homes.

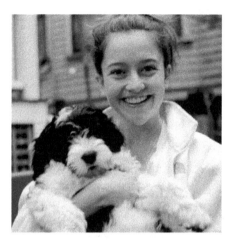

Ellie with Scar

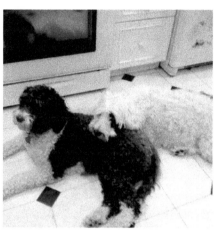

Ezzie and Spray

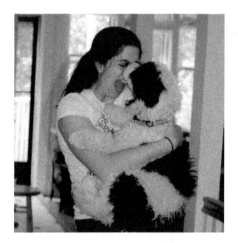

Maggie and Rafiki

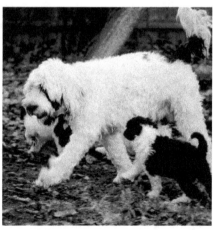

Spray with Zazu

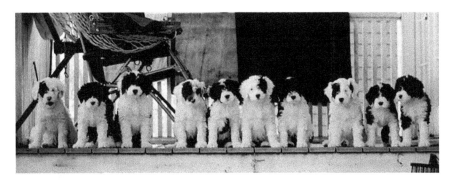

The whole family: Simba, Mushu, Meeko, Sarabi, Esmeralda, Zazu, Map, Scar, Pocahontas, Rafiki (not in order)

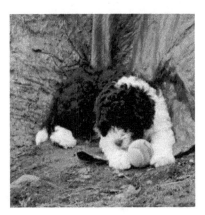

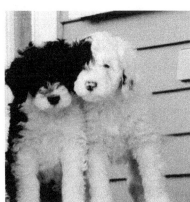

Ezzie

Meeko and Simba

The three original dogs: Splash, Ezzie, and Spray

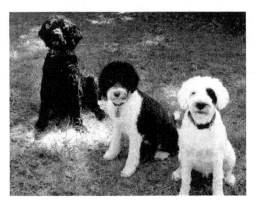

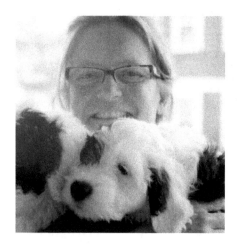

Morgan with Map

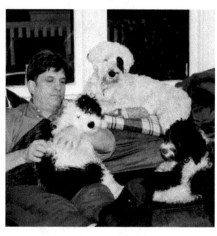

Matt with Rafiki, Spray, and Ezzie

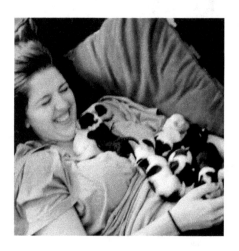

Maggie with pile of pups

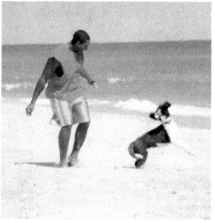

Jay with Ezzie

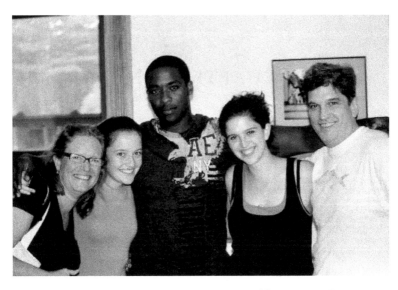

Morgan, Ellie, Jay, Maggie, Matt (from second
move-in day Maggie's freshman year)

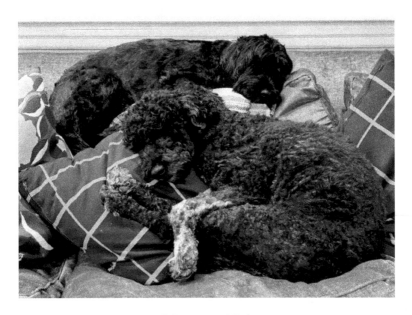

Mayzie and Lily

CHAPTER TEN

The college counselors at Maggie's school warned parents that the summer before college could be rife with disagreements and conflict between parents and teen.

They weren't wrong.

The year leading up to that summer had already contained a lot of goodbyes—nine, to be exact. We had placed nine of Spray's ten puppies in homes in Boston, Cambridge, Arlington, Worcester, and Connecticut. We were happy with the pups' new homes. They were going to be well loved and cared for.

Saying goodbye to Maggie was going to be difficult, especially as I let go of my control over her food allergies. I had protected her and advocated for her for eighteen years. It was time to send her off and trust she knew how to take care of herself.

But I was scared. I had watched Matt—who is allergic to shellfish and various fruit—have reaction after reaction. The first time I saw him crash was at a wedding before we were married. He ate corn that had been cooked with the lobster. He turned gray and passed out. Luckily, respiratory nurses were there as guests, and they dissolved Benadryl in water and poured it down his closing throat. An ambulance took him to the local hospital in Maine. Thanks to the nurses, the paramedics, and the hospital, he was alive to marry me a month later.

Most of his episodes were mild when I drove him to the hospital, but then there were the ones where he collapsed onto the bathroom floor in Cambridge, and on the sidewalk when his blood pressure dropped. These crashes required ambulances.

In Cambridge, while I was trying to get used to the idea that Maggie was leaving, I was also adjusting to having three dogs—something I had never seen in any crystal ball. Splash, Maggie's best friend, was eleven; Spray, Ellie's best friend, was almost three; and Ezzie was still a puppy.

The average age of a Portuguese water dog is ten to fourteen years. Splash, at eleven, still frolicked with Spray, but he had become incontinent and slept a lot, sometimes with his head on my foot as I worked at my desk. Spray and Ezzie wrestled a lot. Ezzie, a curly brown and white PWD, entertained us by running through the living room, hurtling her body over the coffee table and onto the couch.

My mother and stepfather gave me a cherry coffee table for a birthday present the year my mother was sick. It was the biggest gift I'd ever received, and it was the last from my mother, but they were thanking me for taking care of my mother during that last year. Ezzie's nails often dragged across the table during her leaps, filling it with more love.

Ezzie was a busy dog. She nudged her way in if one of us was petting Spray. She needed to be part of the love fest.

While I couldn't believe I had three dogs, Maggie and Ellie didn't find anything odd about it. After all, it was how they grew up. Just as they thought living in an upside-down house was perfectly acceptable.

I excel at comparing myself to others. I have perfected this trait over the years. I worry about how I fit in with different circles of friends—am I smart enough for group A? Wealthy enough for group B? Funky enough for C? Really, the person I'm not satisfying is myself. I've been told over and over by Matt, my daughters, my sister—the baby my mother took to England with my brother and me—that I'm my own worst critic, that other people have better things to do than to spend their time analyzing me.

They're right.

I wanted to raise self-confident girls, who knew their worth. When I listened to them talk about themselves, watched them tend goal or onstage, I saw I had succeeded. They may be competitive when it comes to playing games and driving in traffic, and trying to better themselves at their work, but they don't think less of themselves when it comes to the bigger world picture.

I tried to learn from them.

They are more adventurous than I am.

The three dogs were a backdrop to our lives. We developed a new rhythm with them. The puppies had been at the forefront of every decision we made and everything we did every day for almost three months, but now our dogs became background noise to family events, like getting ready to send Maggie off to college.

We were active, and life was hectic. I didn't miss the little puppies. Even though I often complained when I was super busy, I thrived on multitasking and organizing my time. The busier I was, the more I got done, and the less time I worried about my life at Emerson or home.

Maggie's imminent departure was distracting and emotionally draining, and she hadn't even packed a bag yet. I needed to stay busy to keep that impending loneliness at bay.

At the end of June, after I had finished teaching a summer course at Emerson and Maggie and Ellie finished their film camp, we stuffed the car with bags, a sewing machine, and a bike, and we said goodbye to Matt, who we would see on weekends and for his week of vacation. Maggie, Ellie, Spray, Ezzie, and I escaped to the Vineyard for the remainder of the summer. It was Ezzie's first summer there and the first year we didn't bring Splash.

I was intent on enjoying my last summer with Maggie at home. Even though my mother had died several years earlier, I still missed her running out the front screen door, letting it bang shut behind her, waving her hands and yelling, "Welcome!" when we arrived for the summer. Instead, there was quiet.

We set up in the 800-square-foot guesthouse, which reminded me of playing dollhouse, one of my favorite games as a kid. I could control the family and setting in a dollhouse.

This tiny house was perfect for a family with small children, but as my girls morphed into teens, it became tight. The teeny bedroom Maggie and Ellie shared evolved into a dressing room. Bathing suits, shorts, dresses, and T-shirts lay on the twin beds and floor, and they sprouted out of bags and the built-in bureau tucked in the closet.

Despite the amount of stuff we brought with us, the house never seemed as cluttered and crowded as our house in Cambridge. Often, because their beds were covered in clothes, one of the girls slept in Matt's bed when he wasn't there (before the twin beds were exchanged for a queen) or on the couch in the living room. When Matt arrived on weekends, things became even more snug.

To create an illusion of space, the house had an open floor plan with cathedral ceilings and floor-to-ceiling windows all around. The sun streamed through the windows, infusing the house with lightness. I was more optimistic with the sun.

I was excited about my plans for the summer. We would go to the beach, go for walks, shop in town, and eat yummy meals, like egg salad sandwiches for lunch or potato salad for dinner, and if I didn't want to cook, we could eat at The Galley in Menemsha, where we got burgers and frappes.

But that didn't happen.

Maggie spent more time with her boyfriend, Jay, and other kids her age. She wanted to go to parties. She was trying on new identities, including party-girl.

We fought more than usual—something I had been warned about.

"Don't stay out late," I might have said.

"Mummy, I'll be fine. I'm not stupid. And Jay is with me. Don't worry," she could have replied.

Or...

"I'm too tired to go to the beach today. I'm going to take a nap," she said after working as a counselor at the day camp nearby.

"I thought we were going to go to the beach, and you could nap there," I said.

"I'm too tired."

I knew in my core that some of these disagreements were our way of separating from each other. If I was annoyed with her and she with me, the separating would be easier. But it was killing me. She was already leaving, and I was already missing her.

On the Vineyard, Spray and Ezzie took up space, lying on the couch or sitting in the one armchair. But after living in our upside-down house all year, where I went up and down the stairs to let the dogs in and out of the yard, I appreciated the chance to push open a screen door to let the dogs run outside and take off wherever they wanted to go. There were no fences to keep them in. Unlike Splash,

Ezzie and Spray didn't roam, and they stayed close to home. They slept on the grass outside the door or ran in the field Dads had created with his tractor, behind the big house.

I walked Spray and Ezzie at Squibnocket town beach on the Atlantic side of the island in the early morning, before it became off-limits to dogs at nine a.m. I struggled to get up at 6:15 for my morning walk. But, once in my car, I was awake. The drive never got old as I went down Middle Road, past the Keith Farm where the cows grazed and the view took you over meadows and a pond all the way out to the Atlantic Ocean, and then I drove past the not-yet-opened Chilmark Store. The dogs panted with anticipation.

Ezzie stood with her front paws on the console between the front seats, staring straight out the front window, rigid with excitement, waiting, knowing exactly where we were going.

Standing on Squibnocket Beach in the morning before the sun had yet to burn off the fog, that was my "in the moment time" with the dogs. The dogs ran up and down the beach and leapt into the waves to fetch sticks, particularly Ezzie, who dove into the breaking waves to retrieve them. Spray waited in the swash, then grabbed the stick with Ezzie, as if to say, "See, I helped." The crowds with their coolers, chairs, and towels hadn't descended. The beach was pockmarked with morning walkers and dog people.

When Splash was young, he had barked at birds and humans when we went in Chilmark Pond to row across to a different beach. Spray and Splash followed the rowboat as we made our way across the pond and over the dunes of the barrier beach. Spray wasn't interested in swimming for swimming's sake. She needed a purpose. Ezzie was different. She went in any water, whether it was necessary or not. Big waves didn't frighten her. She dove in chest-first without looking back.

When the girls were at work or out with friends, I started sewing Maggie's going-to-college quilt. I'd had the material for nine months but had yet to even cut the fabric. The dogs, puppies, and college work had taken precedence.

Now, I laid the fabric on the living room floor to cut and pin, though only when the dogs were outside and couldn't walk or lie on my project. Our dogs enjoyed sitting on my quilts while I made them, which was cute but not practical when I was trying to keep the material wrinkle-free. Years later, I made a pseudo-quilt for a dog bed for a future dog to lie on.

To create the feeling of the ocean, I arranged the blues from light blue to darker blue-green. I placed the off-white in the corners to symbolize the foam where the waves crash the shore.

By the end of the summer, right before Matt arrived for a week's vacation, I had made progress on the quilt, but it was far from being finished. I put the quilt away until we returned to Cambridge. This was our last chance to be together before Maggie left.

Making Maggie's quilt took forever. During the pandemic many years later, I created more than a dozen quilts in the same time that it had taken to finish one. Quilting is meditative. It takes me away from my worries. I zone in on the fabric and the sewing. During the pandemic, quilting took me away from the bad news and the longing I had for Maggie and my father—each thousands of miles away—who I missed for a year or more.

When Matt arrived on the Vineyard in mid August, we went to the beach as often as possible. Matt was happiest lying in the sun, then diving in the surf and returning to the sand to fall asleep. Matt can spend hours watching waves crash on the beach, fires blaze in a fireplace, or planes land and take off. Those are his ways to meditate. Ezzie swam with us, and Spray guarded us from the shore.

My sister-in-law, Tia, had been at her house on the island for a few weeks but was preparing to leave. On the night before she and her family flew back to Santa Monica, we gathered at the Homeport, a seafood restaurant in Menemsha, for a goodbye dinner.

Matt and I avoided this restaurant. Their specialty was all things lobster and clams. Why tempt fate? I only ate lobster when he wasn't around. But, we decided if we were really careful and gave the wait staff clear instructions, he would be safe. Matt ordered salmon and broccoli. I had swordfish and corn. None of the offending food was nearby.

Back in the guesthouse after dinner, I was reading in bed when Matt stumbled in from the bathroom.

"I'm in trouble," he said. "Call." His face wasn't as red as it sometimes gets when he has a reaction, but he was having a hard time breathing, which I had only seen a few times. His eyes were wide with fear.

"911?" I asked. "Are you having an attack?"

I pushed one of the dogs, who were lying with me, away.

"Yes." Standing by the edge of the bed, Matt pulled an EpiPen from his bathroom bag and stabbed it into his thigh, holding it there as he counted to ten. As I reached for the phone, he slipped down the side of the bed until he was slouched on the floor.

I jumped from the bed and dialed. "Please hurry. My husband's having an anaphylactic reaction," I said to the dispatcher.

More often, his body flushed red from head to toe, he gave himself the EpiPen, and I drove him to the hospital, where he was pumped full of steroids and antihistamines and was observed for several hours. He always recovered.

This, however, was different. This attack was fiercer.

He stood up, then lurched into the tiny hallway between the bedroom and bathroom and fell again, crashing onto the floor where he lay on his back, dressed only in his boxers.

Ellie was asleep on the couch in the living room. I didn't want her to see Matt like this. She worried about him dying. This would exacerbate her anxiety. There was no way I could convince her he was going to be okay if she saw him. I couldn't convince myself.

Matt and I raised Maggie so she could do whatever she wanted, as long as she carried an EpiPen and didn't eat food if she didn't know where it came from or couldn't read the ingredients. She was very careful, as were we. By the time she graduated high school, she'd had two small reactions. Her pediatrician gave her a Hershey's Kiss right before Halloween when she was about seven. It had an almond in it. We rushed to the hospital, and all was fine. Technically, almonds are more closely related to the stone fruits like peaches and nectarines than tree nuts.

After my mother's memorial service on the Vineyard in 2005, we held a reception back at what had become Dads' home. Maggie mistook the blondies the caterer had made with the ones I'd made without nuts. Again, we rushed her to the hospital, but along the way, we stopped, and as Matt instructed her, she gave herself the EpiPen.

The older she got, the more I had to let go. I couldn't control all the environments she was in. Sending her to a friend's house with a snack and an EpiPen when she was little was so much easier than watching her go out on her own.

But as Matt lay semiconscious in the narrow hallway and I waited for the emergency team to arrive, I didn't want Ellie to see him suffer.

I put the dogs in our bedroom, closed the door, ran to the couch, and shook Ellie awake. Ellie never wakes up. Never. She hated mornings because when she did wake up, someone, usually me, was yelling in her face.

"Ellie! Wake up! Daddy's in trouble. I need you to run to the fire gate and wave the emergency vehicles in." She sat up, her eyes wide open, and looked at me in panic.

Ellie leapt from the couch, pushed the screen door open, letting it slam shut, and bolted outside. But she suddenly returned to slide her feet into flip-flops and ran out again into the dark night. She never asked a question and never looked at Matt.

Later, she told me that she had swatted at bugs, cursed at the night, prayed for her dad, and wondered what was going on and what was taking the emergency team so long. She was angry at being outside, away from her father, not knowing if he was okay. Had she been with us, though, she would have freaked, seeing him the way I did. Sometimes, parents have to take the heat for making what we hope is the best choice in a no-win situation.

Inside, I paced and told Matt everything was okay. I called Maggie. "Daddy's having an allergic reaction. You and Jay should come home," I said.

I neglected to emphasize that this wasn't a run-of-the-mill episode. I don't know if I didn't want to scare her, or if I was trying to trick myself into believing it wasn't that bad. I didn't know when she and Jay would arrive. I didn't know if they were at a party or at the house where Jay lived.

The first responder, a Chilmark cop, arrived within ten minutes of my call. He brought oxygen for Matt, which gave him a little respite. Shortly after that, more cars and an ambulance arrived. The Vineyard has a volunteer emergency service, so most of the EMTs come in their own cars and one brings the ambulance. The vehicles quickly filled our small parking lot and bled onto the grass.

One EMT started prepping Matt for an IV. She asked me to hold the bag of fluid, as she grabbed a towel off the floor to clean off the blood spurting from where she poked him. Her proficiency at administering an IV was questionable. Blood was everywhere. Matt motioned to me and, through the oxygen mask, asked what time it was. He needed to know how much time had passed since the first Epi. Did he need another? More than ten minutes had gone by with no improvement. He wasn't feeling any relief. He still couldn't breathe properly and felt himself slipping out of consciousness again.

"I need another EpiPen," he said through the mask.

"He needs another EpiPen," I told the second EMT.

"No, he's fine," the EMT replied.

He didn't look fine. Matt had been through enough episodes to know when he needed another shot. Later, he said he lay there thinking, *If I die in this hallway, I'm going to be so pissed.*

I called Tia and told her she should meet us at the hospital.

The EMT took Matt's vitals. "He needs another Epi." Matt's blood pressure was dangerously low.

Duh. Just fucking duh.

By this time, Maggie and Jay had arrived. They tiptoed around Matt on the floor, wide-eyed and unsure what to do.

With the second Epi in his system, Matt breathed more easily. He still wore the oxygen mask and was barely dressed. The EMTs covered him with a blanket and hoisted him out of the hallway. After moving some furniture out of the way, with Jay's help, they got him on a gurney, out the door, and into the ambulance.

It took more time for the ambulance to get out of the parking lot—backing up, going forward, driving up on the lawn and finally out the driveway, past Dads in his bathrobe, standing in the front door of his house, staring at the motorcade as it drove by. I followed the ambulance in my station wagon.

Maggie and Jay stayed behind with the police officer to clean up the chaos—the misplaced furniture, the bloody towels from the mess the EMT had made while getting the IV in, and the remnants of ripped paper—so I didn't have to deal with it when I returned. Ellie was still at the gate in her pajamas, so I grabbed her on my way out, and we followed the ambulance for the forty-minute ride to the hospital, not knowing what it meant when it slowed down or the lights came on in the back but fearing it didn't bode well.

He made it.

Matt's stepfather, Bob, and Tia met us at the hospital, and Ellie went outside with GrandBob, where she took comfort in his support. When we were given the all-clear that Matt could go home, Tia took Ellie back to her house. I waited for Matt to be released. It was about midnight.

Just as he was ready to go, he began bleeding internally. Profusely. This presented a new twist. He was readmitted to the ER and then admitted to the inpatient ward, where he stayed for four days. He had painful ischemic colitis, brought on by his plummeting blood pressure when he fell to the floor.

Watching Matt only reinforced how terrified I was of sending Maggie off. Letting go was not my strong suit, and this just made it harder. I had to convince myself I could not only let Maggie go, but I could let go of my fear, too.

CHAPTER ELEVEN

I was torn. I wanted to take care of Matt when he returned to Cambridge, yet with Maggie about to leave, this time with her was precious. Some friends told me kids always came home, and they would always need you, even when they were away. One friend, however, told me she'd never fully recovered from her firstborn leaving home. That sounded more like me.

No matter how prepared I was for Maggie's departure, it was going to hurt, like having a giant boil lanced.

In the end, GrandBob stepped in and watched movies with Matt in Cambridge, while I spent those last few days following Maggie around the Vineyard like a puppy dog.

Matt regained his physical strength after another week at home, and we were able to drive Maggie to Vassar for field hockey preseason.

The evening Maggie, Ellie, the dogs, and I were set to leave the island, Jay drove Maggie to the ferry in his loud VW GTI he had decked out. It rode low to the ground and sounded like a motorcycle when it approached. Ellie, the dogs, and I met up with them in Vineyard Haven. Our car was stuffed with bags and my sewing machine. We were ready to go. Maggie and Jay walked around the docks holding hands. I could only guess what they were saying to each other as I sat in my car, trying to give them privacy. I wondered how their relationship would stand the test of long distance.

They had a good chance, as they had already learned to navigate some big differences between them. Jay was almost five years older than Maggie, which shocked some people, but not Matt and me, and they were learning to navigate the world as an interracial couple. Maggie's heritage is Greek-Dutch-Scottish, and Jay's is West Indian.

Even though most of the campers at the Community Center had figured out they were an item, Jay, who was the director there, was adamant that if someone came upon them in Vineyard Haven, they had to act professional and drop their hands while speaking with them. He took his job seriously and didn't want anyone to assume he was fraternizing with the employees.

Once their goodbyes were done and they reappeared from behind the corner of the Steamship Authority's shingled main building, we drove onto the freight boat. Maggie, Ellie, and I sat in the car on the open deck, watching the moon as we sailed farther away from the Vineyard and a simpler way of life.

Once back in Cambridge, we had two days to get Maggie ready for college. This wasn't a lot of time, but it didn't allow her time to be sad and nervous. I didn't have much time either. We were ripping that enormous Band-Aid off.

I barely remember packing the car. Perhaps because it was too traumatic to imagine my life at home without her? Or because I was too tired? Perhaps I blocked it all from my memory. Somehow, we filled Matt's blue wagon with bags and boxes full of linens, clothes, DVDs, and the egg carton mattress recommended for all college students sleeping on uncomfortable dorm room beds.

Maggie doesn't do emotions. Except when it comes to dogs. And Jay. The most difficult goodbye for her was when she sat on the maroon-carpeted staircase in our front hall and said goodbye to our dogs as she prepared to leave her home. After hugging Spray and Ezzie, she wrapped her arms around Splash, her best friend. "Splashy, please don't die while I'm gone," she said. We all worried about the eleven-year-old dog.

She let Jay put his arm around her, but not me. If you asked her how she was doing, knowing something was troubling her, she answered, "Fine." While I wished she bared her soul to me, I was happy she had Jay.

We didn't speak a lot once we—Matt, Maggie, Ellie, and me—jammed ourselves into Matt's wagon. Maggie fell asleep.

When we passed the rest area a few miles from the Taconic Parkway, where I had stopped with my parents on my way to Vassar my freshman year, I knew we were almost there. In 1976, I was hungover from saying goodbye to friends the night before. And even though my mother was eight months pregnant with my brother, Will, I made her sit in the middle of the front bench seat while the back was filled with my stereo, suitcases, and trunk. I needed the air from the open window.

I had already welcomed a brother into my father's side. Alden was fourteen years younger than me. I didn't see him often as he and his mother, and subsequent brothers and stepfather lived in California. We crossed paths during the summers, and he lived with Matt and me the summer before he too, went to Emerson. After two years, he moved back to where he felt more comfortable – southern California. But, even though I don't see him or his family as often as I would like, when I do, the connection and love is there.

But as an angry and hurt teen, I didn't relish that a baby was on the way. But again, surprises happen. It turned out Will was the best thing that happened. He grew up in a stable home and didn't have abandonment issues. We became a real family when he was born.

Maggie, still asleep in the back, didn't know where we were. It was probably for the best. Sleeping quieted her nerves. Mine flickered like sparklers on a summer night.

As we drove off the Taconic, Maggie woke up, looked around and recognized the shortcut next to a farm on Route 55. She sat up and said, "Stress. Stress. Stress."

Most students don't see the campus at the height of summer when the trees are in full bloom and the fields and quad looks like they have green buzz cuts. The majority of students show up at the end of August and have a week or two of Indian Summer before the trees start to change color to burnt oranges and fiery reds, and the young women begin to wear leather boots. But now it was mid-August, and the trees were still leafy, and the campus grass was thick and lush. There was no hint of the fall to come.

In addition to the athletes, like Maggie, student government types preparing for the school year were on campus as well. The freshmen would join them in two weeks for orientation, and the rest of the student body a few days after that. Until then, the dorm halls echoed in their emptiness.

Our day unloading Maggie and setting up her room went faster than I predicted. She was living in the same dorm I was in my freshman year. The dorm had been renovated, and the room size was smaller. Two large windows looked out over a field called Joss Beach, as it was in front of Josselyn Dorm. Maggie picked the side closest to the door and pushed her bed to line up under the window. We shoved her bureau and desk against the wall.

We were busy running to Target and Bed Bath & Beyond. As we pushed our cart down the aisles, we grabbed a full-length mirror, laundry detergent, and a shower caddy. Shopping usually puts me in a good mood, and shopping with a purpose was extra exciting. There was a reason to spend money—Maggie. She needed all of these items to start her college days well. We were in a race, waiting for the gun to go off so we could start running. Back in her room, I made her bed with the new blue sheets, hung some of her clothes in the closet, and put shirts and pants in her bureau so they didn't just sit in duffle bags on her floor.

I had reached out to Vassar about her allergies, and the school had taken us seriously. First, they asked the incoming class if anyone would room with Maggie, which meant no nuts or peanut butter in their shared space. Tillan Mbindyo said yes. This turned out to be a perfect match. Maggie and Tillan loved movies and TV and spent hours watching and discussing them while eating Wheat Thins. Years later, Tillan read the poem "So Much Happiness" by Naomi Shihab Nye at Maggie's wedding to Jay.

The All-Campus Dining Center (ACDC) at Vassar was also receptive to Maggie's needs. Two dining hall administrators gave Maggie, Matt, and me a tour of the center, pointing out the various stations: salad, cereal, hot and cold foods where Maggie could find safe food, and the stir fry station she should avoid. One of them opened a refrigerator door, and I saw mini tubs of cream cheese inside.

I squeezed back my tears. "Look, Maggie. Do you see?" She could eat her favorite bagels with cream cheese safely. She didn't have to worry about cross contamination from the huge vat of cream cheese kissing the one full of peanut butter.

Back at the dorm, Matt said, "We should think about going."

I wasn't ready. Maggie wasn't either. Maggie excels at packing her feelings into boxes with lids only she can take off.

We had finished the sweat-inducing move. We had carried her life—clothes, books, blankets, sheets, and towels—up the stairs in the August heat from Matt's wagon. She stood on the wide steps of her dorm waving and looking over her shoulder after pushing me away from hugging her. The best I could do was wave back.

I would be back in two weeks for freshmen orientation, which calmed me a bit. I could meet her roommate, go to the parents' orientation, and most importantly get to see Maggie again. None of that helped. According to Ellie, I still cried all the way home. That's three-and-a-half hours of crying.

CHAPTER TWELVE

Maggie was gone. She would never live at home again, in her room with the light blue trim and the poster of Johnny Depp and Orlando Bloom from *Pirates of the Caribbean* and the photo of the Patriots snowball game they won in 2003 or the poster of the movie *Ladder 49*, which her uncle had produced, and the fuzzy blue rug my mother had given her when she was nine. But I kept her room the same for visits, complete with stuffed bears and dogs, until years after she moved to L.A. Then, I turned it into my sewing room. Her desk held my sewing machine, and one of her cabinets concealed all my fabric. When necessary, her room also made a great guest room with a Victorian walnut double bed from Matt's family. But those days were far off. After she left for college, I couldn't remove a crumb or piece of lint off the floor. The room had to remain Maggie-centric.

I wanted her back.

I had to let go and to try to do so gracefully, if you call stalking graceful.

In my home office, where student papers piled up waiting to be edited and graded, and the bookshelves were overloaded with memoirs, I spent hours on Facebook waiting for Maggie to log on. I never said anything. I didn't let her know I was monitoring her online presence, but when her name flashed on the screen, I could imagine her in her dorm room. We never engaged and she didn't post photos a lot, but I was grateful she had agreed to let me be a Facebook friend.

Matt and I returned to Vassar two weeks later, bringing Ellie and Jay with us. Ellie didn't want to lose Maggie, her go-to person, and Jay wanted to see where Maggie was living and spend as much time with her as possible.

This time, the campus hummed with activity. Screaming upperclassmen welcomed the freshmen class and their parents. The environment had shifted from quiet to boisterous. Cars parked on lawns; noise was everywhere. Maggie's roommate, Tillan, had arrived, and life at college had really begun.

So too, had my separation.

We left the three dogs at home with Scott, who lived in Somerville, one town over. At home, the dogs adapted to the new family configuration better than I did. Spray constantly showed me how to be a mom. She had not only let her puppies move to forever homes, but she had also encouraged it. I couldn't let go the way Spray had.

We planned to return on weekends to stand behind the fence and watch field hockey games, but seeing her play field hockey wasn't the same as having her live at home. I knew this day would come, ever since I had dropped her at daycare, gone to a back window and spied in to see how she was doing. She was playing with a friend. Not missing me.

But those weekends wouldn't start for another month or so.

In Maggie's dorm, we organized her room some more, pushing beds and bureaus around, and we commemorated the move-in by taking pictures of Maggie and Tillan, Maggie and Jay, and Maggie and us. As festive as we made the occasion, my stomach felt as if I had just dropped several floors in an elevator. I wanted to stay, help the girls with their room and meet more kids on their floor, but it was time to leave for the second time. This leaving thing was not getting easier.

I had done my best as a mother. While I made mistakes—it's impossible not to—it's learning from our mistakes that's important.

I had to believe Maggie was going to be okay. Unlike Spray, who had pushed her pups from her nest, I was pushing and pulling back at the same time, probably sending mixed messages to Maggie. I wanted her to live an independent, exciting life, but couldn't she do it in my backyard?

We said our goodbyes for the second time, and I climbed into our wagon with the Patriots logo on the back window. Ellie and I sat in the back, while Matt and Jay, with his long legs, sat in the front. I cried for about an hour this time, which was an improvement over the first goodbye. I was wearing sunglasses, and Matt only realized how disheveled and distraught I was when he turned around to look at me—or had he been peeking in the rearview mirror all along? Matt reached behind and patted my leg.

Jay asked, "Are you crying?"

"Yes, but if you tell her, I'll kill you," I said.

I didn't want Maggie to worry about me. I wanted her to focus on her new life and the adjustments she was going to make, not the ones I was making at home in a quieter house, at a kitchen counter with one fewer for dinner every night.

I didn't know then that Ellie, Matt, and I would form new

routines. We ate out more often, mostly at Full Moon around the corner. They had the cheesiest macaroni and cheese and large, soft French fries. We ate Chinese often, because we didn't worry about Maggie's allergies and the issue of cross-contamination with sesame or nuts. We watched *Glee* and *Grey's Anatomy* with Spray and Ezzie on our laps and Splash on the floor.

While I was preparing syllabi for my fall writing classes at Emerson, Maggie was at field hockey practice twice a day and trying to keep up with freshman orientation activities.

Several days after our final goodbye, she called from Vassar Brothers Hospital. This was my worst nightmare—my family members dying from their allergies.

"I'm okay," she said. "I have some sort of pneumonia. But I'm fine."

I didn't know what to do. Maggie said she was "fine." I didn't believe her. Should I rush back to take care of her or let her manage on her own in her new, independent life?

"You should go," Matt said. "You're her mom. Go." While my classes hadn't started up, Matt's work at the airport prevented him from leaving.

Even though my classes hadn't started, my courses' syllabi demanded my attention. But Matt was right, I was more flexible, plus I wouldn't be able to focus on my work while I was anxious about Maggie. My daughter had pneumonia. I drove the three and a half hours back to Poughkeepsie to find Maggie still in the hospital with the two students who had brought her to the emergency room. They were watching *Say Yes to the Dress*, ironically one of Ellie's favorite shows, while waiting for takeout Japanese food to be delivered.

Considering how sick and exhausted Maggie was, she was in good spirits. After being discharged from the hospital, Maggie and I went to Alumnae House, the campus inn across Raymond Avenue from her dorm, where I had reserved a room. She stayed with me for three nights, sharing my queen bed. We were cozy. I was sad she didn't feel well and worried about her, but I also reveled in my chance to take care of her one more time.

While the rest of the freshmen ran around, getting to know the campus and each other, Maggie and I split our time between Alumnae House and Baldwin, the campus infirmary. Occasionally, we returned to her room, for her to touch base with Tillan and new friends in her hall. I left her alone for a couple of hours, and when she got tired, I picked her up, and we returned to Alumnae House.

I bought her course books in the campus bookstore, just like I had bought mine thirty years earlier, and every morning I brought her gooey cinnamon rolls from a local restaurant, Baby Cakes.

I didn't know when to leave.

During one of our visits back to her room, when no one was there, Maggie broke down. "I hate this. I hate college. I want to go back to high school," she said between sobs.

Great idea! I could put her in the car and bring her home. But, of course, no matter how much I wanted to have her back, I encouraged her to buck up.

"Well, I'm not sure this year's seniors would be too thrilled at having you back. It's their turn now. It's your turn to do this," I said.

I left the next day in my 2001 blue wagon with school stickers affixed to the bumper and back window. It was not new anymore, like when I had taken my mother to doctor appointments five years earlier. Back then, the clean car smelled of leather. Now it bore signs of age and hard work, years of protecting and carting around a family with dogs. The front seat was ripped, sand crusted in the seat crevices. Remnants of food embedded the flooring.

I left with a giant hole in my heart, but after that, I rarely heard another word from Maggie about being homesick. I could always tell when she was, however, by the tone of her voice when she called me in Cambridge. Ellie told me later that Maggie occasionally called her to say she was missing home, but she didn't want me to know because she didn't want me to worry. She knew breaking up our foursome was going to be hard on me. She was right.

On one weekend visit home, Maggie caught herself referring to her dorm as "home," and looking at me, she quickly said, "I mean, my room." I had read enough essays by my Emerson students to understand the conflict they felt between school and home—and if she was calling school "home," it was a good thing. She was feeling comfortable there, and I was happy for her. But I'd be lying if I didn't say it stung.

When she was home—at our home, where she had grown up—I followed her around like one of our dogs, just like on the Vineyard. It was an art I was perfecting. If I could have attached myself to her with Velcro or a leash, I would have.

Later in the year, her high school asked me to be on a panel to talk to current senior parents about what the freshman year is like for parents. Ellie said, "You'll be good at that, Mummy. It's really hard, and you did a great job." I wasn't sure I agreed.

I sat on the panel, along with the school psychologist, and told parents, mostly mothers, how they had to let their children go and let the kids contact their parents when they wanted. Parents could watch them from afar. Their faces fell. One mother came up to me after. "How long did it take to get used to her being gone?"

The joke is that if parents do their job well, they'll win first prize. Their children will leave them.

My mission, once my daughters started to depart, was to figure out who I was without the title role of mother. What were my supporting roles? What could I develop more, now that I had more time for me? I had not been the mother who took vacations without her kids. I had not been the mother who worked full-time. I admired those mothers who could draw the line between their lives and their children's, but that wasn't me. The line between my life and my children's had been drawn in the sand and washed away.

While being a mother is probably the most important role of my life, it might not always be the most time-consuming one. My assignment was to figure how to spend my time—teaching, working with ceramics, sewing, or spending more time with my husband, like I did before kids.

That fall, the mornings were quiet, as I had anticipated. Maggie didn't wake up, blast The Fray and One Republic on her laptop, and carry it around the third floor, into the bathroom and back into her room. Ellie, however, took that habit over pretty fast, playing Katy Perry, Taylor Swift, and Sarah Bareilles. I even missed Maggie's clutter, her backpack in the middle of the living room, and her boots strewn across the front hall.

Only three people sat around the kitchen counter for dinners of my roast chicken and meat loaf or Matt's spaghetti, meatballs, and homemade tomato sauce. The door to Maggie's room stayed shut. I didn't want to peer into a void. I didn't hear conversations or fights break out between the sisters. The energy and noise level had diminished. Even the dogs seemed less energetic.

Those were the hard parts in adjusting to a new family unit. The fun part was spending more time with Ellie and not feeling torn between the two girls. I drove Ellie to school when it was my carpool day. We listened to a lot of female pop and top-forty. The other kids in the carpool, especially one of her cousins, got sick of hearing Ellie and me belt out, "Do you ever feel like a plastic bag..." along with Katy Perry. Besides singing in the car, other favorite times were watching *Say Yes to the Dress* and random HGTV shows, like the *Property Brothers* and *Fixer-Upper*, after her homework was done.

I continued to feed the cast and crew before Ellie's performances in high school and sold tickets to eager parents and grandparents to the shows. By the time Ellie graduated, she had been in about fifteen plays, including *Paradise Hotel*, *Esperanza Rising*, *Merrily We Roll Along*, and *The Rimers of Eldritch*.

Suddenly I dreaded the approaching years when Ellie would be gone as well. How would I fill the spaces these departures created? Would walking the dogs be enough? Maybe I'd have to find a new career to keep me out of the house five days a week.

To fill the immediate abyss, I signed up for a ceramics class and a dog training class. Matt and I planned a yard sale. I did physical therapy twice a week for what might have been a herniated disc in my spine. I drove the carpool and taught my two classes—magazine writing and creative nonfiction—at Emerson. While I was focused and engaged in an activity, I couldn't ruminate on Maggie's absence. I couldn't imagine what my life going forward might look like when I was teaching Ezzie to sit and stay, or centering a lump of clay on the wheel.

Doing ceramics or quilting forced me to pay attention to the project I was working on. Everything else—all my anxieties and loneliness—fell to the side. I couldn't drift away on a missing-Maggie cloud. My bowl would be off center. I didn't miss Maggie at the studio. I held the ball of wet clay on the wheel, maneuvered it into a centered position, then pulled, opened, and looked into what I hoped would become a bowl.

Some of the other potters at the ceramic studio asked why I was back again after a few semesters away. My answer in my "happy" voice was, "I'm giving this to myself as a present, now that I don't have as much to do at home. It's the start of the empty nest for me." Really, working in clay offered medicine to prevent me from falling apart.

My hobbies—sewing and ceramics—gave me tangible objects as a result of the work I'd done, which was quite different from teaching and writing, or being a parent, where the end products were either longer in coming or nebulous. Students came and left. Every semester I welcomed a new batch, and every semester I had to say goodbye. You'd imagine I'd be an expert at goodbyes, considering how many years I had taught. But I wasn't.

I wasn't going to get depressed. I knew the signs that preceded a full-on depressive episode: the lack of energy, the sadness, the loneliness, the loss of self-worth, not eating, sleeping too much. I was determined not to let it happen again.

CHAPTER THIRTEEN

I didn't need to read the inventory of symptoms the CDC and NIMH listed as those associated with depression to know I felt like shit. But I read it anyway. The list includes:

- Ongoing feelings of sadness, guilt, or hopelessness
- Loss of interest in things you once enjoyed
- Significant changes in your sleep pattern, such as trouble falling or staying asleep or sleeping too much
- Fatigue or unexplained pain or other physical symptoms without an apparent cause
- Problems concentrating or remembering things
- Changes in appetite leading to significant weight loss or weight gain
- Physical aches and pains
- Feeling as though life isn't worth living, or having thoughts of suicide

I checked off every item on the list. Yup, all those symptoms were mine. Depression and being sad are easily confused, but they are different. Sad is hard. But depression is like draping a wet blanket over your head, and it's so heavy you can't pull it off. Women are also twice as likely as men to suffer from depression. In 2010,

I was one of 11.4 million adults (eighteen and older) to fall into a depression canyon.

I had a hard time explaining to friends or family why I was depressed. Depression doesn't always have a reason.

From an objective standing, there were many reasons why I shouldn't be depressed. I loved my two daughters, my husband was smart and funny and loved me, I had a nice house, I had a decent career and three challenging but entertaining dogs. But loss made me unreasonable, and depression didn't listen to the rational side of an argument. It took hold of the irrational and felt ensnared by a thorny bush, so after a while, it was the only side I could hear.

I listened to the internal voices screaming at me that I was fat and lazy, I didn't contribute to the family financially enough, I was inefficient as a teacher and writer, and I was pathetic as a mother and wife. I didn't find joy in anything. I didn't quilt. I didn't play with the dogs. I didn't have any affect. I was empty, like a flat cutout character standing in a movie theater.

Matt was supportive. He tried to reassure me that I wasn't the waste case I thought I was. I came up with a nickname for myself: FLODOUGH. *Flo* for flop in life, *dough* for being fat. We used that code word for years, but it slowly died out over time, for which I'm grateful.

There were, of course, no facts to back up any of those assertions. Depression is an excellent liar, and it's hard to see that when you're drowning in its lies. I received positive evaluations semester after semester, and in 2013, just before Ellie left for college, I was honored with Emerson's Alan L. Stanzler Award for Excellence in Teaching. Matt, Ellie, and GrandBob came to the ceremony in one of Emerson's theaters with students and faculty in attendance. I bought a new outfit for the occasion, a matching top and skirt, but was sure I looked like a bag of potatoes when called up to the podium.

My department chair, who had nominated me (twice), was there to cheer me on. An administrator who introduced me also reported that students said I was honest with my critiques, sometimes too honest. She then turned the mic over to me. I spoke about how much I loved my students and how important their voices were, and that I had enough belief in Emerson that even my daughter was attending.

This was an enormous honor and validation for all the work I'd done, but when depression visits, it's hard to rationalize with it or shut the door on it. Even when I felt okay, the door was always held open a crack with a doorstop—like the embroidered brick of my grandmother's. At any moment, the door could fling all the way open with a kick of a foot.

During previous depressive episodes, I watched from above, appalled at how angry I got. I was irrational. In my twenties, when I had lived in a basement apartment, I hit a wall so hard with my fist, the framed quote about finding self-respect that my grandfather had shared at a Yale commencement fell to the floor, and the glass shattered. My mother had this quote calligraphed for all her children upon graduating from our high schools. The crash made me even angrier at myself.

As a wife and mother, I yelled at the kids and Matt when I sank too deeply. I got irritated when they messed up the kitchen or didn't help with the dogs. I got mad at myself too. I hit my head with hardback books, pummeled my legs with my fists, and controlled myself enough that I didn't headbutt walls like I had in my teens. I was so embarrassed by my behavior, I didn't even know how to apologize for it. If I could wish for anything, it would be for a rewind and to have a do-over of those experiences. Shake the Etch A Sketch clean.

Given my past, my therapist and I were rightly concerned about how Maggie's departure might affect me.

I didn't like relying on medicine. I wanted to be better by my own willpower. I wanted to get with that program of my mother's. Matt was eager for my therapist to jump in with help. But, I believed I could manage on my own, without medicine. I wasn't going to be weak and dependent.

Clearly, I was wrong.

I didn't separate gracefully from those I loved. But I was adamant I'd be okay. I just needed to stay busy. If I was active, I reasoned, I wouldn't have time to dwell on the things that made me sad. I still had Matt, Ellie, and the dogs to focus on.

I even had prepared for how panicked I might feel during Maggie's last year. I didn't want to experience everything as a last— her last play, her last field hockey game, her last time celebrating her birthday with friends, the last family ice skate at the school rink.

I had asked a photographer I knew from other photography sessions to take pictures of the girls when Maggie was in eleventh grade and Ellie was in eighth. I planned it carefully. If I waited to take them during Maggie's last year, I'd probably cry. This way, it seemed random—just beautiful black and white photos of my two daughters standing and sitting together, totally random. Little would the viewer know we were in the middle of Mount Auburn Cemetery. Full of trees and bushes and flowers, it provided the perfect backdrop for the photos. No graves in sight. Maggie and Ellie hugged, lay on the ground together, smiled at each other, and then we stuck me in one as well to give to Matt for Father's Day.

During most of our fall weekends, we went to Vassar. Jay came with us if he got time off from Best Buy, where he excelled at selling high-end TV and home entertainment systems. He was one of the best in the country, winning third place regionally for Magnolia Home Theater in the President's Club one year.

We visited Maggie several times in September and October, always leaving the three dogs behind with Scott. We went to all her home games and stood in the stands cheering for the Vassar Brewers.

In September, we wore baseball hats advertising Vassar Field Hockey and sunglasses to shield ourselves from the baking sun. By October, we wore fleece and hats to keep warm. We made friends with the other parents who came out for the games. The players had a loyal following. We also traveled to the away games at Western Connecticut and The University of Scranton. Future years had more away games.

Maggie was the backup goalie to a senior goalie for the first half of the fall semester. But halfway through, the coach started Maggie, and in her second game against Union College, she made eighteen saves versus the three Union's goalie made. Vassar lost to Union in a shoot-out, but Maggie had made a name for herself. That game turned everything around for her. She was the starting goalie for the remainder of her Vassar career. Articles were written about her, and she took her role seriously.

Maggie was making friends with the other players on the team, some of whom were in her wedding years later, and she and Tillan spent hours together watching movies. Life was settling down for her.

Maggie was focused in the goal, despite the loud cheering. She came out of the net to cut the angle down when an opposing player charged her. She saved balls with her stick; and with her humongous leg pads, she kicked balls away; and she slid to the ground, protect-ing the net with her whole body. My stomach and nerves couldn't always take watching her in goal. There was so much pressure rid-ing on her, and this mama bear wanted to protect her.

Matt and Jay learned some Vassar chants, including one about beer. "Heineken, Michelob, Miller Light, Let's Go Brewers, Fight, Fight, Fight!" The team was called the Brewers because Matthew Vassar—who founded the college in 1861—had made his fortune as a brewer. When Vassar's doors opened, 353 women between the ages eighteen and twenty-four walked in. When Maggie started at Vassar, the student population, both men and women, was about 2,450 students.

Vassar was the first women's college with a Phi Beta Kappa chapter and was known to be comparable in rigor to men's colleges. In 1969, Vassar turned down an invitation to merge with Yale and went co-ed instead. In 1976, both Matt and I entered as freshmen.

While Matt wasn't new to chanting at Maggie's games—he'd perfected his cheering at Maggie's high school games—Vassar parents, players, and coaches weren't prepared for Matt's booming voice from the sidelines. For a guy who isn't particularly social and liked spending time at home, he bellowed across the field without shame. When Jay accompanied us, the two of them could whip the fans into a vociferous chorus.

On a sunny, warm September weekend with no field hockey on the calendar, Matt and I decided to have a yard sale. We covered the front porch, steps, and sidewalk with items to sell from our base-ment, mostly a few odd wedding presents, such as one candlestick, from twenty-two years earlier.

We didn't need the Nordic Track we had inherited from my mother and Dads when they downsized. We had never used it, not even for a tie rack. It sat in our basement for years, reminding us each time we were near it that we should really start working out.

This was the year we were going to get rid of it. Not too surprisingly, no one bought it. We left it there at the end of the day, and it went in the garbage truck on Tuesday.

The kids were young the last time we'd had a yard sale. We sold baby items and toys they'd outgrown. Since then, the junk in the basement had blossomed. Not only did we have twenty years of boxes of clothes, an old foosball table, furniture, sleds, toys, and housewares, but Matt's aunt Eilie had also lived in our little apartment for four years, and when she died, her furniture from her home in DC also took up residence in the basement.

Ellie displayed a lot of her toys at the yard sale: Groovy Girls and their accessories, and Barbies and their accoutrements. We let her keep the profits from anything she sold. One woman dickered with her over the prices, complaining that Ellie hadn't marked her items at yard sale prices.

Ellie's response? "Then she doesn't have to buy them."

Fortunately for Ellie, another woman bought a lot of the toys for her granddaughter to play with when she visited. Years later, Ellie missed those Groovy Girls. Letting go of your past can be heartbreaking, even when you know it's the right thing to do.

The sun heated up the sidewalk. Old college friends who had recently moved to Cambridge stopped by, and at one point, I looked up the street and saw Zazu and his owners marching down the block. They must have seen our yard sale advertised on Facebook.

I hadn't seen him since he left us in April. I yelled, "Zazu!" Our neighbors across the street heard me. They too had loved the big Zazu when he'd lived with us and came out to greet him, as well.

Zazu regally pranced down the street, with his head held high and his body swinging out behind him. He was a gentle giant. We took him and Ezzie into the backyard, and he stood still while Ezzie leapt around and over him. Zazu had inherited Spray's calm demeanor. Ezzie had not.

I wanted to wrap my arms around him. I was so proud of him and happy and sad at the same time. I still thought of the puppies as mine, but they weren't. I had to respect that Zazu belonged to someone else. He had moved on. Just like Maggie.

Later in the fall, as the days got shorter and darker, I started dog training classes with Ezzie on Thursday evenings in the gym of the local armory, a few blocks from our house. While it was still warm out, Ezzie and I walked. Actually, she walked me, pulling me the whole way. But once the cold weather set in, I got lazy, and we drove the half mile.

Initially, Ezzie and I went alone, but as the year progressed and my mood disintegrated along with the weather, Ellie joined us. While Ezzie and I practiced our routines of sit, stay, or down, Ellie sat on the bleachers along the wall, reading, doing homework, or watching. Her presence calmed my anxiety, and I didn't feel so bereft. Perhaps it was unfair of me to drag Ellie into my moods, but my desperation was mounting, and she was a buoy I could cling to in the rocking ocean.

Orange cones divided the room into four sections, each de-voted to a specific level of training. We started in Level One, where Ezzie learned to walk on a leash, sit and stay. Ezzie's brown hair was often floppy, which endeared her to the teachers. One trainer said, "You should put her hair in barrettes or a pony so she can see."

Ezzie was a model student and passed Level One without much difficulty. We graduated to Level Two, and eventually even to Level Three, where she learned to "leave it."

Ezzie enjoyed class so much, she even learned to roll over and jump. But at home, Ezzie forgot her manners. Spray had taught her some of her good traits—like sit and down—but she also taught her how to jump at the glass window in our front door. She charged the front door with her mother when visitors arrived and leapt at any and all family members out of sheer joy and exuberance. Eventually, we protected the window from shattering with a sheet of plexiglass screwed onto the doorframe.

The humans who lived in our house and those who visited were not particularly fond of the leaping. Every time Ezzie jumped at us with her mouth open, she naturally grabbed onto something—a scarf, a bit of jacket, or an arm. She often clawed us as well, leaving scratch marks on our legs, which later turned into bruises.

We filled a basket with stuffed animals and trained her to "get a toy" when we were at the door. In reality, this meant we yelled at her from outside, "Ezzie, get a toy! Go get a toy," and then waited until she did so before coming inside. Holding a toy in her mouth meant she was less likely to jump. Instead, she just squealed and turned in circles like her mother.

I don't make a lot of money teaching. Luckily, Matt had good benefits from his jobs. We added my income to his, but if I had had to live on it alone, it wasn't going to happen. The higher education system is broken. Adjuncts, like me, do most of the teaching, and while we may excel at our jobs, it's the name brand that pulls students in, so the tenure track professors all look great on paper, and some really are fabulous teachers.

Without a book to my name, I had no chance of moving up. So, I sometimes thought about leaving teaching, but whenever I searched the help wanted ads or thought about other alternatives, I always returned to the classroom because my students engaged me. That may sound like hyperbole, but I liked developing relationships with them, getting to know what their interests were and what challenged them. They were like giant puppies, each one unique—some with energy to burn, some quiet and reflective. I have worked with students who have profiled interesting characters in Boston, and I have worked with students who write essays about their health, homes, and families, and their experiences with sexual abuse.

The students usually bonded as they shared their personal narratives. I facilitated the conversations. I avoided micromanaging them, and students learned to trust their voices and their peers' comments as the semester progressed. They also learned the value of revision as I mandated it in all my classes.

Teaching when the girls were younger had afforded me the time to be with them and write for a variety of newspapers and magazines.

But teaching college students the year Maggie left tested me. Maggie and Ellie had always been younger than my students. They were always developmentally separate, and I could share funny kid stories with my classes. Now, Maggie had caught up, and when I looked out into my classroom, I saw lots of Maggies.

When students talked about their weekend activities—the parties they attended and the drinking they did—I wondered what

Maggie was doing. If they wrote about missing their families or not missing their families, I saw Maggie in their essays. When I witnessed how stressed and tired they became as the semester wore on, I worried about Maggie and her workload.

As the fall season progressed, I got used to saying goodbye to her at the end of the weekends, sort of. We developed a rhythm in those months, but when October ended, and with it the field hockey season, so did our routine.

The only contact I had with Maggie after that was through Facebook and the phone calls she made as she walked on campus, a habit she shared with other college students. The calls came randomly when she strolled between classes, or from a meal back to her dorm. She always hung up abruptly when she reached her destination. She was ready for the next activity. I was not.

Parents often have to play catch-up to their kids. Maggie's mood may have been sad when she hung up, leaving me to worry about her. But by the next phone call, she could be bouncing with enthusiasm. I was exhausted following along.

This was Maggie's way of signaling that maybe she was missing us the way we were missing her. But she never came out and actually said so.

All of our contact happened when Maggie wanted it. If I reached out to her, she was often too busy to talk. I didn't want to seem like the needy mother I most definitely was. So, I continued to stalk her.

Every time I signed on to Facebook, sitting at my desk tucked away behind the TV room in my home office, where no one could see me, I felt like a teenager with a crush. I immediately checked to see if she was on. When I saw the green circle next to her name, my heart beat a little faster. If the circle didn't show up, I was disappointed. I rarely engaged her in conversation; I just liked knowing she was there. I missed Maggie. I missed our old family.

Matt didn't talk much about missing Maggie, but he missed watching movies with her, cooking for her, and going to the Patriot football games with her. He started watching more of them at home with a dog for company instead.

Maggie came home at Thanksgiving. She was happy to see the dogs, particularly Splash, who was still with us. When she came in the door after her ride left her at the front door, she dropped to her knees as the three dogs rushed her. "My friends." She rubbed their backs and took their licks in stride.

During the weekend, she played with them, running around the backyard with Ezzie and Spray. She also slept a lot. I didn't see her as much as I had hoped because she was beat, and when she was awake, she was doing homework or hanging out with Jay, who had come in from Marlborough, where he lived with his parents and younger brother. I once again followed her around like one of the dogs. She did find time to sit at the kitchen counter and play cards—gin and double solitaire—with me.

The actual Thanksgiving meal was festive. A crowd of more than a dozen people crammed around our table, and Matt did most of the cooking. He really is the better of the chefs, while I baked a fudgy chocolate cake for dessert, something I excel at.

When Maggie left at the end of the long weekend and I returned to the classroom, I saw a dazed look on my students' faces—the same look Maggie probably had on hers. It said, "Oh no, I didn't get as much work done as I should have, and now it's crunch time until the end of the semester."

Despite being stressed with a load of papers to read and edit, I appreciated the distraction. There wasn't time to focus on Maggie.

Then I was into my Christmas shopping. I took pride in finding fun gifts for family and friends, like the boots I got Ellie one year, or the books I gave Maggie. The Christmas madness of shopping, decorating the house, and baking cookies helped me ignore how easy it was to disparage myself for only having two kids instead of three, for not making more money, for being an adjunct, for being too fat, for struggling with money—to spend money, not save money. I wasn't organized, I didn't keep a tidy house, I didn't know how to cook, I ate too many sweet things. Concerned voices from my mother and stepfather swirled in my head. I tried not to listen. My own voice was loud enough. I compared myself to everyone. I set ridiculous standards for myself I'd never be able to achieve.

I started crying.

I cried if someone was nice to me.

I cried if I was alone.

I hid my self-hate and feelings of being a loser under my bed with the off-season clothes and beach towels. I didn't want anyone to know how bad I felt. I didn't want to ruin the holiday spirit.

Maggie had left, Ellie would leave, dogs would die, and my mother had died, which meant my father and stepfather would die too. I was a burden to my family, especially my kids. I didn't want to harm them any more than I already had. I was so worried about any permanent damage I could do to them. Mothers were always to blame. I had not escaped scar-free from my own birth family.

I couldn't and didn't know how to talk to friends and family about how bad my mood was. Who would understand? I didn't want to be an inconvenience. I didn't want anyone to worry about me. I had to be fine. I had to. I had to push through and be okay.

Eventually, I couldn't keep my crying hidden. I couldn't laugh or smile. I was scared to leave the house. I sat on the green couch in the living room with Matt one afternoon, sobbing, shaking, and holding his hand like a life raft. I wanted to peel the skin off my body. "I can't stand this," I said. "I can't do anything right anymore. I'm losing my mind. I hate myself."

"Stop," Matt said. "You're fine. You are a wonderful person." He tried to put his arm around me. This was not effective. I was staring into the Grand Canyon of failure and ready to jump.

If I did go out and drive, I wondered what it would feel like to drive off a bridge or hit a tree. I knew I wouldn't do those things, but the ideas were there. Did other people have those thoughts?

Matt suggested I call my therapist, who prescribed an anti-anxiety medication to get me through the rest of the week. Before we could get the prescription filled, Matt gave me a Xanax left over from an old prescription of his. I saw why people liked Xanax. My jitters came to a halt, and I could let go of Matt's hand and consider going outside. I learned later that my therapist wasn't a fan of Xanax. Apparently, it was addictive. I could see why. Ativan, which she prescribed for me, was also effective but had a somnolent quality to it, which made working and interacting with others a challenge during the day.

After Christmas, my therapist suggested antidepressants. I was a failure. I couldn't keep it together through work and stamina.

I didn't like being on medication. I didn't like the inevitable side effects—dry mouth, low sex drive, weight gain, sleepiness—and I didn't like that this dark cloud in my head could only be controlled by artificial means. What did it say about me and my strength of character if I couldn't control it alone? My mother had always used the old "pull up your bootstrap" idea when any of her kids were down. I couldn't even hold on to the bootstraps, let alone pull them up.

Sitting in my therapist's office on the second floor of her garage/ office in Newton, twenty-five minutes from my house in Cambridge, I tried to convince her I was okay.

"I just need to stay busy," I said.

From behind her desk, she said, "I think we should try older antidepressants. I don't think SSRIs are helpful for you."

I had tried Wellbutrin, Effexor, Prozac, and Zoloft. I gained weight and fell asleep a lot, especially when I was driving, which was not ideal. I dozed at red lights, and Ellie had to nudge me awake when the light turned green.

"I'm worried I have Epstein Barr virus again," I told my therapist at one meeting, a year before Maggie left.

"Why? It's unlikely," she said.

"Because I fall asleep driving a lot. Today, I thought a car moved from a parking space, and I jerked my car to avoid it. But the car hadn't moved."

She sat up straighter. "It's the Prozac. We need to find you something else."

I went off my meds but didn't share that with my family. I'm not sure why. It wasn't until I crashed at Maggie's departure, that Matt learned of it and got angry at me.

"Why did you do that?" he scolded me. "What made you think that was okay, and why didn't you tell me?"

I was experimenting. I wanted to see if I'd be okay without meds. I was tired of being dependent on them. I wanted to be strong enough that I could power through. I wanted to be a bouncy, cheerful, successful, optimistic person.

After Maggie left, I also wasn't honest about the severity of my collapse.

Even the dogs couldn't make me smile. Ezzie always made me

laugh as she charged for the couch and leapt over the coffee table. Often she used the coffee table as a launching pad, and her nails put scratch marks on it.

When my mother was diagnosed with small cell lung cancer in 2005, I took an immediate leave of absence from teaching, and Dads and I took care of her. I became my mother's advocate in the hospital and their chauffeur, driving them to and from Dana-Farber Cancer Institute in what was then a four-year-old blue Volvo wagon, which I loved. It was safe, clean, and new, not like it was years later. The wagon outlasted my mother by thirteen years and ran more than 150,000 miles.

That wagon lived through my children's childhoods and then some. It took dogs to the beach for early-morning walks on the Vineyard, it took Ellie to school and back in carpool, it took both girls to soccer games all over Eastern Massachusetts. It collected Cambridge parking permits on the back-left side of the wagon and Vineyard beach stickers on the right side. Ellie once stuck a bunch of random stickers on the bumper and back. Three of them were from The Green Room, a clothing boutique she worked in after graduating college and performing in Vineyard Playhouse productions.

One night, when Matt was more frustrated than usual, he said, "Why don't you call Susie?" He hoped another voice would help.

"She doesn't want to talk to me." Not only did I know Susie through Cinemaze and the Vineyard, but I also knew her through Jay. Jay and her younger son, Asa, became best friends because they spent a ton of time together building Legos when Jay's mom was taking care of Asa. Not only did Asa and he hang out in Cambridge, but Jay also started spending summers with Susie's family because his mother worried about summer in the inner city. Thus, Maggie and Jay met working at the Community Center as counselors on the Vineyard.

"Just try," Matt pressed me to call.

I called and Susie picked up, even though she was at a restaurant for dinner with family. She talked to me for a few minutes. "This is a passing phase. You do have friends. You'll be okay, and I'll call you later," she tried reassuring me.

When I started crying more frequently, Maggie, who was now home on winter break, and Jay tried to lighten my mood by taking bets on how often I cried each day. First, they had to agree on a definition. Did welling up count? Or did tears have to fall?

In the kitchen making chocolate chip cookies, a favorite pastime of mine, I cried when thoughts about Maggie returning to school after vacation interfered with taking a cookie sheet out of the oven. Baking had always been a cathartic release for me but could only distract me for so long.

"Look, she's crying again," Jay said to Maggie one night while I was at the sink washing dishes.

"Any tears?" Maggie asked.

"No, I'm not," I argued as I turned my back to face the sink and the dirty dishes. "I am not."

I smiled, listening to them debate whether I was crying or not. But I couldn't control the invasive thoughts about Maggie leaving or how Ellie would leave in three years, or being an adjunct instead of a full-time professor, or not going to the gym enough, or not walking the dogs every day. Something always made me feel worthless.

I remained adamant that I needed to stay busy, as I had in the fall—I needed to find more activities to occupy my time. But the thought of all I had to do to keep myself busy exhausted me.

No matter how many friends told me you never really lose your children, that you're always a parent, I knew Maggie had left home for good. Even if she were to come back to live with us, it would only be as a visitor. There would be no more Saturday soccer games or church on Sunday mornings or homemade Halloween costumes of dolphins, unicorns, princesses, and clowns.

CHAPTER FOURTEEN

Before turning forty, I could hardly imagine myself at older ages, but suddenly, after I crossed the line to fifty, I started to imagine what my life might be like at sixty and even seventy. I could almost touch it. Matt and I started talking about our future—a different kind of future than the one I imagined my children were envisioning for themselves. They were looking forward with lots of open doors. I was imagining what I wanted to do before I died. There were more closed doors for me. I was too old and didn't have the funds to go get an MFA. I would never be a full-time professor.

As they wondered where they might live, what they might do professionally and with whom they might live as life partners, Matt and I talked about where we might retire and how we would support ourselves.

We still lived in the same house we had brought our babies home to. Maybe, we thought, if the kids moved to L.A. (with Maggie in the film industry and Ellie as an actor), we could live there part-time. Maybe we could still have an adventure as older people, even as we started to tie up loose ends while Maggie and Ellie moved forward in their lives.

During a Christmas visit five years earlier, my mother had listened to me worrying about what my life was going to be like as I approached fifty. Sitting in one of my armchairs by the fire, she said,

"My fifties and sixties were my best years, until my back started hurting."

This was before she was diagnosed with the cancer that took her life eight months later, when Maggie was thirteen and Ellie was ten.

I revisited that conversation frequently, when I worried about being lonely after the kids left. Her parenting trajectory had been different from mine. She had had four children—me, her first child, when she was twenty-two and her last child at forty-one. I had my two children in my mid-thirties. I missed my mother's advice, even when I didn't want to hear it.

She told me I was doing a good job of being a mother and working, but she was also good at making me feel I wasn't doing as much as I could, and that my house was messy. She was always busy, and I inherited that trait. I don't know how to relax. I'm always taking on a new project—either for myself, like a quilt, or helping someone else out, figuring out how one of my daughters can move their careers forward.

I don't stop. I don't rest. Rest is overrated. My mother hardly watched TV or movies. She considered them a waste of time. When she was sick, however, she actually started watching *Everybody Loves Raymond* and movies distracted her. I also gave her lots of books.

As the spring semester loomed, Maggie returned to Vassar in mid-January, without any breaks in sight until spring vacation in March. Field hockey was over. Our routine of weekends on campus, where Matt and I also reminisced about our time there—in the campus bar and at a dance party his house had—were done until the next fall.

It snowed and snowed and snowed. I sent Maggie photographs of the dogs in the backyard, romping in snow deeper than they were tall. Ezzie leaped through the snow the same way she jumped through water, with a high arch to her back. I sent Maggie pictures of snow piles in front of our house, making her guess which ones had cars under them.

During a hard and fast snowfall, the city fell silent. The streets and sidewalks looked fresh and clean. Then reality set in. Snow was a nuisance. I walked in the street most of the time because the sidewalks weren't shoveled, or the pathways were so narrow they were hard to navigate. I couldn't see around corners when driving because the mounds of snow were so high. People's moods frayed.

I should have paid more attention to the warning signs, acknowledging them as they crept into view, but I didn't want to believe it would get me again. I was stronger and super clever. I could outfox it this time. I ignored the crying jags, the anxiety building inside, and the feelings of inadequacy.

But depression won.

Winter on the East Coast was defeating me. While not officially diagnosed, Matt and the girls were convinced I had seasonal affective disorder (SAD). I definitely have to work harder in the dark months to stay out of depression's depths.

Visiting L.A. to see Matt's dad and his sister's family in the middle of winter was a treat full of sunshine and warmth. When the kids were little, Matt took them out for their spring break, and I joined them when mine overlapped. The break in the weather was welcome. The sun on my face and on my back when I walked the park by Tia's house was like unwrapping a long-awaited Christmas present.

Depression had hit me before, mostly during times of transition. It didn't take a rocket scientist to trace this back to when my father put my mother, siblings, and me on that Pan Am flight when I was nine.

When I felt like crap my freshman year, I was clearly depressed. But, no one really called it that then. But I sure didn't feel great. I didn't have the energy to go to class or do my work. Any enthusiasm I could dig up was designated to drinking and smoking pot. I might have been having fun, but really, I was numbing my feelings. I visited a counselor at the building that housed the mental health resources, where I checked off the boxes on a sheet: do you feel hopeless, do you lack pleasure in the things you used to like, has anyone in your family died by suicide? I hovered over this question. Yes, I finally checked. My grandmother when I was very young.

In addition, I was already anticipating my mother and stepfather starting their own family as I left their home.

My mother had delivered her first three children early, and Will was no different. I happened to be home during October break when he was born. When I came home from a night out with friends, I found a note on the stairs from my stepfather: "Gone to Hospital."

I visited my mother the next day. I brought Will a stuffed dog, much like the one my mother gave him. They were a pair. He named them Orange and Brown, and he still has them, sitting on a shelf in his home office.

When he came home from the hospital, I visited him in his bassinet. I looked in at the swaddled being and said, "I should hate you, but I can't. You're too cute." He was an innocent bystander, like the ones in drive-by shootings. I didn't need to target him. He didn't bring this on himself. He had done nothing to hurt me. In time, I fell in love with Will. One of the reasons I moved from New York to Boston after college graduation was so I could get to know him.

Sometimes random people got confused when they met us. The gas attendant asked, "How old is your baby?" The Christmas tree salesman told Will, "Go help your mom, sonny." And even as adults, people can't quite figure out if I'm a grandmother, sister, or even a weird wife.

As adults, we are close, even though eighteen years separate us. He was fourteen when Maggie was born; I was fifty-three when his first daughter, Clara, was born.

But at Vassar, before marriage and kids, my grades slipped, and my mood continued to decline. I decided to take a leave of absence my second semester. That sounds so simple and smart. It wasn't. I was a mess. I don't even remember how I decided. Leaving my friends behind and leaving a plan behind was brutal. But maybe I just knew that things would be very bad if I stayed.

I lived at home, saw a psychiatrist twice a week, worked as a hostess in a Harvard Square restaurant, focused on becoming healthy again, and got to know my baby brother. I didn't want to hate myself.

But, I wasn't in control of my emotions. Depression was. It's a terrible way to feel. I knew, intellectually, I shouldn't feel the way I did. If I could pull myself out from its grip for a minute, I knew logically I couldn't be that bad, sad, or dumb. But a depressed brain doesn't let you feel the rational way. It digs a hole and fills it with little, tiny beach pebbles. They look so pretty and tiny on the sand, but once you start packing in the hole, it gets heavier and heavier, until it's hard to ignore.

The emptying nest and snow were quite a combination, and it hit me hard.

Some parents reveled in their newfound freedom—going out to dinner, traveling, not worrying about their kids all the time, having fun. That wasn't me. I missed Maggie, and knowing Ellie would be leaving soon didn't help. I wondered what my purpose would be if it wasn't to take care of them.

A clinical diagnosis doesn't exist for the empty nest syndrome, like there is for depression, but there should be. Parents should be warned that this might hit them. They should be prepared with distractions. They should have friends at the ready to guide them through this phase.

I had devoted so much of myself to my children that with the imminent departures of my kids, I questioned my identity.

Depression was an out-of-body experience—I didn't own my body or my emotions. I hated that I couldn't manage or explain what was happening to me. I was stuck; I couldn't move forward or backward. The quicksand had a hold on me. I looked at the half-finished quilts lying around the house, including Maggie's. I couldn't go near them. Every time I pictured Maggie at school, I broke down, mostly behind closed doors in my office, where no one could see me. I sat at my desk, staring at a blank screen on my computer as tears rolled down my face.

"What are you doing, Mummy?" Ellie asked from behind my closed door.

"Working. I'll be out in a minute."

I didn't want her to see me and feel responsible for making me feel better. I knew Matt was aware something was askew, but I was trying hard to buck up as much as possible. I worried he was frustrated with me. Ultimately, I think he was frustrated he couldn't help me.

I slept, cried, and berated myself for all the things I didn't do well—being a mother, a teacher, a wife. I couldn't lose weight. I didn't have friends. The list was long. The reasons didn't necessarily have to make sense to anyone other than me. I trudged through each day like flypaper, and flies were collecting on my body, sticking to me, slowing me down even more, hiding the real me. I felt like everyone was staring at me, judging me.

During previous depressive episodes, I had gotten angry at myself and my family. The triggers for these events were not as obvious as this one. When the kids were young, I could get overwhelmed, ironically, taking care of them. Matt wasn't around as much. As a reporter and then-editor at *The Globe*, he was often at work past dinnertime. The girls and I got used to our routine of eating without him and talking about all things girl: periods, boys, sex.

When he changed shifts and could be home for dinner, Ellie said, "Now we can't talk about vaginas anymore."

"What do you want for dinner?" I asked the kids every night. They could choose between my homemade chicken nuggets, my meatloaf, cheesy chicken, or macaroni and cheese. I excelled at kid food—my homemade chicken nuggets were a favorite. I sliced a boneless breast of chicken into chunks, then soaked them in milk before breading them. I fried them in olive oil, and the kids and I ate them up. Matt got the leftovers.

But teaching, freelancing, being a mom, and worrying about the health and safety of Matt and Maggie, and eventually Ellie, sometimes was too much. Living with the idea that one of them could die in an instant because of something they ate was terrifying. It was like a low cloud hanging over me, just waiting to dump rain.

One night when the kids were young, I started to lose my cool, crying and getting mad at how much I had to do and how little control I had on my life. I took my keys and drove away from the house and let myself into my parents' condo on Memorial Drive in Cambridge. They were on the Vineyard full-time and only used the condo when they were in town for doctor appointments, theater, or music.

The condo was on the sixth floor with a view of the Charles River and Harvard's athletic field on the Boston side. I ran my hand along the wall, looking for a light switch. Turning lights on in this condo was not as automatic as it was at home. I didn't belong there the way I did at home, where I knew where everything was, including the light switches.

I didn't go in the kitchen or the living room. I didn't open the fridge or sit on the sofa. I went straight into the second bedroom with twin beds we called "hammocks" because the mattresses were old, worn, and sagged. This room was also the resting place for my grandmother's dollhouse she had gifted me when I was about twelve because I loved dollhouses. Not only could I control the family in a dollhouse, but I also enjoyed the interior design aspect. Setting up a room with miniature furniture, books, and food allowed my creativity to flow. This translated later to my quilting.

My grandmother had bought it for ten cents as a young girl, and it still included some of the original furniture, such as the wicker sofa and chairs for the porch. For my senior project in high school, I "renovated" the house. I glued new wallpaper in the bathroom and bedrooms, and I coated the exterior with a mixture of sand and paint to look like stucco.

I lay down on one sagging twin bed and slept on top of the covers. I didn't want to disturb my mother's order in the condo. They were never aware of my night visit.

When I woke in the morning, I drove back to my own home and family. This was not one of my proudest moments. Ellie, in particular, was freaked. "Please don't do that again," she said as we sat in the kitchen. "Please don't leave."

I never did.

This time, when the empty nest and my purposeless future

loomed ahead, I didn't run away in the same way. I just hid and cried—running away in another way.

I was much more anxious. This was new. Anxiety surprised me. Little bugs crawled inside my skin, trying to eat me alive. Depression was an old friend, like a comfortable blanket. Depression was debilitating. Anxiety made me crazy. I wanted to shake myself hard so the bugs would fall out.

I'd been anxious before, for specific reasons—before a test or teaching the first class of the semester—but this time, I was anxious all the time. I was afraid of going outside and of being left alone at home. The anxiety was paralyzing. I wanted to rip my skin off, in hopes that I could rip out the anxiety with it. The only activities that calmed me were petting Ezzie and Spray, sitting with Matt on the couch as he reassured me, and wrapping myself in blankets while lying on the sofa or bed.

"You'll be fine," Matt said as he held my hand. "You're okay. Just take a deep breath."

I obsessed about death. I wanted to live long enough to see Maggie and Ellie graduate from college, get married and have children, if they wanted them.

I began to appreciate how difficult it was for Ellie's anxiety. I had assumed you could talk yourself off the ledge, but not so. Just like depression, anxiety isn't rational, either. You can't just tell it to go away. You need coping skills, good friends, and medication. Only then will it begin to listen to you telling it to get the hell away.

Depression is also embarrassing. At least it has been for me. No matter how much the general public has become more aware and accepting of mental health issues through celebrities' struggles, I still felt a stigma and shame associated with my struggle. I heard my mother's voice. Why couldn't I just pull up those damn boot-straps? I hated those bootstraps.

Friends and colleagues are more comfortable talking about their sore throats than their mental health.

It takes more than a pep talk to get through a depressive jag or an anxiety storm. But knowing I had friends and wasn't alone did provide comfort. You have to learn which friends to turn to and how to ask for help.

I worked hard not to be hampered by depression. Ellie worked even harder to weave her OCD into her life in a way that didn't prevent her from having a successful life. Ellie particularly thrived as an actor onstage. "I'm someone else when I'm up there," she said. Onstage, she focused so hard on her work, the anxiety and OCD just fell to the floor.

Offstage was harder.

I didn't know about OCD or depression as a child. I was introduced to both later in life. OCD is a crippling mental health disorder, and I was proud of Ellie. She was one of the most self-aware people I knew, who worked hard to quiet her OCD voices. She did have compulsions—tapping and counting—but as she got older, she was able to manage them better.

There are OCD tendencies, which my mother had, such as keeping an insanely spotless home. There should have been velvet ropes forbidding visitors from entering her rooms. On the Vineyard, she didn't allow anyone to eat in the TV room, but my kids figured out a way around that. They sat just outside the doorway on the stairs with their food and watched the TV from that vantage point. While my mother thrived on control, she probably didn't have invasive thoughts that kept her from living a fulfilling life.

Regardless of how much I cognitively understood that depression and anxiety are actual illnesses, I still felt weak of nature. I believed a pump-up session should work, like an exercise session helps you get stronger. If I had a stronger character, I figured, I could pull myself through this time in my life and get on with it. Didn't other people? Sometimes it felt like I was wearing a sandwich board announcing my depression. I didn't like how my illness and, consequently my behavior, affected Matt, Maggie, and Ellie. They worried I would hurt myself.

"Mummy, promise you won't hurt yourself," Ellie asked numerous times throughout her childhood. "Yes, I promise," I assured her. But, I also thought they would be so much better off without me. No more fights, no more compromises. They could live life without my handicaps getting in the way.

I did eventually reach out to some friends—virtual friends on Facebook. They were safer than the friends around the corner or across the street. I didn't want to bother my friends. I couldn't describe what I was feeling. I didn't want people to worry about me. I just wanted to crawl into a cave. Reaching out on Facebook reminded me of sitting next to a stranger on a plane or bus, where we exchanged life stories without judgment or concern. My traveling partner could forget me as they disembarked from the plane or walked away from the bus. I was a story, not a friend.

I posted a request on Facebook asking for reading material.

"Does anyone have any suggestions for light reading to distract me right now?" I posted.

I was astonished by the response I got. I compiled a long reading list that successfully distracted me from my worries. Books like *The Guernsey Literary and Potato Peel Pie Society* and *The Postmistress* were a great diversion late at night in bed.

CHAPTER FIFTEEN

One Saturday in February, Matt and I drove to Ellie's fencing tournament at St. Sebastian's School in Needham. Ten schools met up to fence one another. Parents brought food and water for their teams. Usually, I was on top of my game, contributing something to eat and drink. I was an excellent soccer mom/fencing mom, but under these new circumstances, I focused simply on getting to the meet. I was even known for yelling at the coach on the opposing soccer team when Ellie might have been eight. I almost got Ellie thrown out of the league. But now, just getting to the tournament was challenging enough. I wasn't even embarrassed by my lack of contribution; buying water was beyond my capability. I just didn't care.

Despite how crappy I felt, I wanted to see Ellie compete. I tried hard not to let my moods compromise my mothering. I wasn't always successful. This day, I considered it a success that I had gotten out the front door and into the car. Matt drove.

Once there, the jitters started. Instead of talking with other parents about their kids and the event, I hung back, sitting high on the gymnasium bleachers. I didn't want anyone to see how incapable I was of having a conversation.

Ellie was in the center of the gym with her teammates. The fencers were dressed in white, like chefs, and wore masks over their heads and faces for protection and carried their weapon of choice. Ellie used an epee. Epees have a bigger guard than foils, but sabers and epees differ from foils in the way they are used. You slash with the saber, while opponents poke at each other with the foil and epee.

Sports were not Ellie's thing. She spent most of her time in the theater department at school, taking classes and acting in as many productions as possible, but she was required to play one sport a year. She tried basketball her freshman year, and now it was time to try fencing.

The fencers moved around the gym from bout to bout, so I followed Ellie from one event to the next. In one round, she fenced students from Maggie's old school. I sat in front of some parents who were talking about their kids and classes. Some were reading the school newspaper. I wanted to jump in and tell them Maggie had written for the paper, and I had been a parent on the Parents Association, and I was an alum. But I didn't. I wasn't sure of how appropriate it would be, and I couldn't find my voice. I focused on Ellie instead.

As soon as her bout (or match) ended, I walked away in tears.

Matt found me and stood in front of me as a shield as I faced a corner of the gym, so no one could see me cry. I depended on him so much. I didn't want him to burn out. I knew there were times when he was frustrated and just wanted to shake me and tell me to get a grip, the way I wanted to tell Ellie to stop worrying about everything, but mental illnesses have their own bouts with rational thinking.

Finally, my therapist convinced me to try Nortriptyline, an older antidepressant from the tricyclic family. Nortriptyline was stronger than the others I had tried, with equally powerful side effects, including dry mouth, constipation, and my favorite, weight gain. It was approved for use in 1964, compared to Prozac in 1987. I also had to have my heart and kidney functions tested periodically. The therapist was hopeful it would pull me out of the deep despair I had slipped into. I hated the intense dry mouth. It felt like cotton balls were wedged in my cheeks. This was not handy when I was teaching, and my mouth was glued shut. Water bottles became my friends.

Once depression seeped into my bones, veins, and arteries, it was a constant companion. Some times were easier than others, but it lurked, waiting, ready to pounce like our puppies—but this springing wasn't fun and playful. This feeling hurt and lingered.

Although Maggie used to call my medicine my "happy pills," antidepressants don't magically make patients happy. At least they didn't for me. They just brought me back to a level where I could begin to function and feel like I was me. My problems didn't magically disappear. I still had the same issues I'd always had—feeling abandoned, insecure about my success in life, scared of confrontation—but now they couldn't overwhelm me.

Slowly, I got tougher. I stopped crying all the time. I got out of bed in the morning without a struggle. My urge to rip the skin from my body ceased. I didn't feel like such a burden to my friends and family. Maggie checked in periodically from school to see how I was doing, and I continued to talk to friends on Facebook and in real life.

While I gained some of my sanity back, I also put on almost twenty pounds—a lovely side effect, which didn't thrill me. I was embarrassed. I wanted to pin a sign to my chest that announced why I had gained weight, but clearly that wasn't an option. I couldn't win. I got to choose Door 1: depression or Door 2: being overweight. Awesome. One of my Facebook friends, an old friend from my single days, told me to weave ribbons through my red hair, and I'd look great. The weight gain, like the dry mouth, stayed with me for years.

How quickly we judge each other, whether someone is overweight or smacks their dry lips together. I reminded my daughters that everyone struggled with something. Some people are more private about their struggles, but no one gets through life free.

While I was functioning better, my depression still squeezed itself into my daily life when I least expected it, like a sucker punch. As I sat in my doctor's office during one appointment discussing the chronic pain in my right leg, tears ran down my face for no apparent reason.

My uncle, my mother's brother, called me one evening after hearing I was in a difficult place, and just hearing his voice say, "Hi, Morg. I heard you're having a hard time," on the phone set me off, and again, I couldn't control my crying. Knowing someone cared, someone who was a "grown-up," who I looked up to, respected and loved, made me feel safe.

My sister tried to bolster me with supportive phone calls, but she had been kicked in the head and stomped on by a horse and was dealing with a severe head injury. She needed her own support system. Had I not been depressed, I would have jumped in, carting her to doctor appointments and organizing her care—something I'm good at doing—but it was all I could do to phone her. My mental state was precarious, so I only visited once.

I found solace in my classroom and with my dogs: Splash, Spray, and Ezzie. Watching Ezzie and Spray wrestle in the living room brought me joy. They jumped on each other, ran around in circles, played tug of war, or chased each other in the backyard. They took turns lying on their backs, batting at the other, mouthing a neck. When they tired of their games, they curled up on the back of our couch, flattened our cushions, and kept me company while I napped or watched TV. Spray had moved on from her mom days, although she and Ezzie had a close relationship and often groomed each other in the house and during car rides with Scott. Splash was happy when he found a comfy spot where he could lie down and not be bothered by the ruckus the other two were creating.

Like the dogs, teaching turned my focus onto the moment, not looking backward or forward. I was in the classroom twice a week for two classes each day. I dreaded going in, worried about my dry mouth but also whether I could find enthusiasm for my courses.

But my focal points became my students and the material. At home, my focus bounced around, but the students needed my attention. The classroom provided a reprieve. I concentrated on my students' questions and their writing. Their energy swept me up. We talked about story ideas, sources, and how to engage a reader as fast as possible. I was exhausted after class, but during those two hours, I stopped obsessing about what a bad person I was. For those hours, I experienced real relief.

I was lucky and grateful Matt and a few close friends hung in there with me. Susie and Laura U. called frequently to make sure I was okay. I wasn't hooked on exercise yet, but I later discovered that working out with my cousin, Betsy, and a trainer a few times a week was excellent medicine for my depression. If I could work out, I could do anything. I got stronger and kept at it for years.

I wasn't a great conversationalist when I was depressed. I didn't have much to add to any topic, and just contemplating how to contribute to a discussion drained my energy. I sat at Susie's dining room table in her large brick Cambridge home with a cup of coffee in front of me. I sipped my coffee, and eventually, I opened up and talked about my mood.

"I just don't like myself much," I told Susie and Laura U. "I don't think I have much to offer anyone."

My friends tried to reassure me and even tried to relate their own struggles to mine. But in my deep pit of depression, I couldn't truly hear them. I wanted to stay at the dining room table, but I also wanted to run and go home to hide only a few blocks away.

My friend Lisa invited me out to dinner one night. We went to Casablanca in Harvard Square. The restaurant was smaller than it had been in my twenties and thirties. It was one of the first places Matt and I had gone on a date—upstairs at Casablanca, where I had talked about my future plans. I was studying for the GREs and wanted to pursue a terminal degree (I had an MA) to become a full-time professor. Matt, it turned out, was impressed with my independence and drive. We returned there years later with his mom and stepfather, where we talked about writing. I was working on a novel that didn't ever go anywhere, and his mother, a sociologist, was working on a book about blood sacrifice that was published posthumously by the University of Chicago.

I had nothing to say to Lisa in the smaller restaurant. I twisted my napkin in my lap and pushed the food I couldn't eat around on my plate. "How is Jackie?" I asked Lisa about her daughter. "Does she like school?"

"She's great. Making friends."

"What is she studying?"

I have no idea what she answered.

I couldn't wait to return to my home, a hideaway where I didn't have to pretend to be okay.

Social outings were torture, even with friends who might care. Talking about feeling shitty and not wanting to be around anymore isn't lively conversation. I didn't want to saddle anyone with my worries and, honestly, I didn't even know how to describe what I was going through so others might understand. I wasn't sad. I was in a mire of despair. I wasn't frustrated by work or being a mom. I just wanted out. I didn't want to feel so lost and hopeless.

I understood why people took their own lives. I got it, but it made me sad. Matt told me suicide was selfish. I didn't agree. I didn't know how to tell him I could relate. I didn't want to scare him. I also understood how hard it was on the survivors. My father's mother had ended her own life when my father was in his twenties. He doesn't talk about it much, but how could that not have affected him?

Unless you've been significantly depressed, it's hard to equate it to anything someone else can relate to. I really believed that my family would be better off without me. I wasn't being selfish about suicide. Suicide would end the pain and relieve my family of a tiresome responsibility.

One day, when Ellie and I were sitting in the TV room with its red walls, Ellie muted the volume and said once again, "Mummy, promise me you won't hurt yourself."

"I promise," I said.

We turned back to *Say Yes to the Dress* and delved into the fantasy world where we picked apart the dresses. We were not fans of Pnina Tornai, a high-end designer. Some of her dresses were elaborate and beautiful, and others looked like high-class underwear.

My depression followed me wherever I went. At book group, I sat silently, trying to pay attention to the discussion around me.

I had been in this book group since I returned from Pittsburgh in 1989. My cousin, Betsy, invited me into it. Many of the original members had gone to elementary school together. As time went on, people moved or dropped out, and it became smaller and more intimate.

At book group, we spent a lot of time sharing our challenges, with our children and spouses. Everyone had something, but why would anyone want to hear from me? I stayed quiet. I didn't want them to know how far down I had sunk.

I was afraid much of the time. Afraid of myself. Afraid of the world. Afraid I wasn't strong enough to fight this invisible monster consuming me.

I didn't tell anyone at Emerson what I was going through. It didn't occur to me that it might be important, or any of their business. The only time I let my personal life infiltrate work was when my mother had gotten sick and I asked for an immediate leave of absence. The chair at the time granted it without question but did ask I teach the first day until they could find a replacement.

It had been easier to ask for help when my mother was sick than when I was depressed. People are uncomfortable talking about their mental health. I'm not sure why, but I was the same. If I'd had a broken leg, I would have asked for help. Perhaps we think we can pull ourselves out of mental health struggles, that mental health issues reflect on us in a negative way, that we are weak and can't handle life's challenges.

Obviously, that isn't true. But the stigma is there.

One day, I bumped into a full-time colleague as we crossed the intersection of Tremont and Boylston.

"Can I ask you a question?" I asked as we dodged students and cars and got to the sidewalk safely.

"Yes."

"Do you think it's okay for me to use one of my own essays to demonstrate how to approach a particular concept?" I wanted to show the class an example of when showing, not telling, was beneficial.

"You are the expert," she said, as we squeezed our way through the student traffic between classes.

Months later, when I was feeling better, I saw the same professor outside of her office near my cubicle, which I had hid in when desperate.

"Thank you for your encouraging words a few months ago," I said. I looked around to see if anyone else was listening. "I wasn't doing so well then. I'm much better now, but I was dealing with a mood shift."

"I know," she said. "I'm glad you're feeling better." That was it.

I wondered if my students could tell I was off. I didn't know if my dry mouth puzzled them or if my anxiety permeated my lectures. Would they worry about their teacher the way I worried about them sometimes? That wasn't their job, and I didn't want them to.

Plenty of students, over the years, had disclosed their issues to me, whether it was their depression, anxiety, sexual abuse, death of a loved one, learning differences, or family emergencies. Matt and some colleagues doubted the veracity of the students with dead relatives, who asked for extensions, but I always accommodated them.

I understood them. That is one of the reasons I loved teaching college and was good at it—I didn't want anyone to suffer or feel alone the way I had at college and, if they did, I wanted to help them put the pieces together.

I had been one of those students. I sat in the back of the room, didn't talk, and often skipped classes. How ironic that I now stood, or sat, at the front of the same kind of classrooms. I didn't let the students off the hook though. Even students in emotional upheaval needed to be held accountable. Those expectations also helped ground the students, just as my work—editing and grading the papers—helped me. The structure in my life—whether teaching, taking classes, or training Ezzie—kept me from slipping further down the drain.

After dabbling in different jobs, including hotel management and advertising, I applied to graduate school for writing. As a graduate student at Emerson, I was assigned to teach Writing About Literature, an introductory overview of short stories. Back then, Emerson was housed in brownstones in Boston's Back Bay. Classes were held in former living rooms and bedrooms. I lived in a group house in the South End before restaurants moved in and the place became gentrified. It took me twenty minutes to walk the half mile to school the first day. I've always said, if I walked any slower, I would be walking backwards. I entered that classroom with dread, not excitement. I had been the kid in the back of the room, unable to raise my hand to speak in class. Suddenly, I was in front of the class, and my job was to talk. I was getting paid to talk. I couldn't slink out of this one.

I spoke in a monotone and didn't look any of the students in the eye. But I did it—I taught the class. At the end of the semester, a student came up to me and said, "You got better, you really did."

More importantly, I discovered I liked it. So, I did it again, and again, and again. For more than thirty years.

I wanted the students to engage with the material I shared; I lived and worked in the moment, focusing on the students in front of me, much like my dogs focused on what they wanted in the moment. My mind couldn't wander to my anxieties and worries. I focused.

In my winter of despair, I worried about Maggie and Ellie. They worried about me. I struggled with guilt, knowing I was the cause of their angst and Matt's. He still says he doesn't like to read about it. It was one of the worst times of his life. That makes me so sad and guilty. If I could have done things differently, I would have. I hate feeling responsible for one of his worsts, even if no one is truly responsible when the depression curtain drops.

I wanted my family to focus on their lives. I didn't want my mental health to distract them.

Even though I knew separating from my children—Maggie first and eventually Ellie—was the right thing to do for them, and for me, that didn't mean it wasn't hard and painful. Years later, my therapist said it was hard for me to separate from the kids because I wasn't sure I was good at many things. But I knew I had been a good mother. I doubted that while depressed, but once healthy with perspective, I was confident about my mothering.

She was right.

But in 2011, Maggie continued to call regularly to check on me. Ellie was with me all the time, and I could see how my moods could upset her. I didn't want them to feel responsible for cheering me up, which was difficult to do anyway.

"Please don't worry about me," I told Ellie, who didn't look convinced. "I have an illness, like your anxiety. It will pass. I don't want you to be concerned."

Ellie had a hard time letting go of that concern.

"I'll be fine, Ellie. Stop worrying." Did they hear me? Was I a constant concern?

I appreciated their support more than they'll ever fully know, but parents shouldn't depend on their children too much. Even as they grow older, children still need to be children, and parents still need to be parents. Role reversal is hard on both sides.

During my mother's months of illness, I was terrified of what my life would be like without her. I relied on her as a mother, friend, and grandmother. I couldn't imagine my life without her. After she died, I was often caught off guard by a photo of her on a shelf in my house; or when I went into J. Miles, the boutique we loved, I almost expected her to be with me. The smell of new clothes and a clothing steamer, and seeing clothes that reminded me of her, always made me stop, remember, and miss her for a minute.

Shortly after she died, I went into Porter Square Books, and the smell of new books, one of my favorite smells, got me. Tears sprung from my eyes before I had a chance to check them. I didn't shop with my mother here; why was I so upset? Finally, I understood. The last time I'd been in was to find books to read to her.

One day, during the year she was sick, I had reached out to her as we were going into her condo after a trip to the hospital. "I'm scared, Mummy," I said.

"I can't help you," she replied. "Go talk to Matt about this." That was that. Her role as my mother had vanished. Fear took over.

A few months later, Matt and I hosted my whole family— Dads, my mother, and my three siblings—over for dinner. My mother cried at the dining room table. "I'm going to miss so much," she said. "You're all going to talk about me when I'm gone."

I didn't want to push my children away. I wanted to always be a mother to them, but when the depression was at its worst, it was hard to remember that. Fear, pain and unhappiness, I've learned, can change your behavior even if you don't want them to. On the other end, I had to be patient with the one who was struggling, whether it was with me or someone else. I couldn't snap my fingers and have everything back the way I wanted. Getting better was a process.

I wish I had woken up one morning a changed person—one of those perky, upbeat, *look on the-bright side of life* people who always have something positive to say about everything. That didn't happen. I'm not that person, and, honestly, sometimes those people are just too much for me to bear. Do they have problems, insecurities? Do they just bury them in a deep underground tunnel?

Climbing out of a depression is slow—it's a few steps forward and then a quick slide backwards, like in the movie *Homeward Bound*, when Shadow, the older dog, falls into a hole and tries to climb out of it, as he and his dog and cat companions are making their way home after being separated from their humans. He keeps slipping backwards and tells his buddies to go on without him. But with a cheering section above the hole, Shadow keeps trying, and after a few false starts, he gets out, although viewers don't know that for a while. The suspense is a killer.

With Matt, Maggie, Ellie, and my friends rooting for me, I kept at it, and over time, I got out of my hole. Matt said he could tell when I was back and was glad to see me. I laughed more. I danced around the house. I played with the dogs. Ellie and I watched more TV. I stopped asking him if he regretted marrying me. I went outside without looking over my shoulder. I started working on Maggie's quilt again. I sent it before March break. I didn't collapse at the post office or a bookstore. I ate and I read.

I didn't trust feeling better, however, convinced something would derail me. What if I took on too much work? Would Ellie's upcoming high school graduation send me running? Would Matt have another life-threatening allergic reaction? Could I keep my daughters safe?

Despite those fears, I managed to move forward. Part of climbing out was learning to reframe myself, to recognize that my world was changing. I needed to like myself, with my bumps and curves. My children were separating from me. The time had come for me to get a grip. This didn't happen overnight—it was an ongoing challenge.

I never understood the commandment "Treat thy neighbor as thyself." Why would any neighbor want me to treat them the way I treated myself? I reserved the best for my kids, Matt, my students, and friends. I had heard the refrain, "Don't be a show-off," or "Don't be bad," frequently in my youth. If I started to acknowledge how well I'd done on a test, or sewn a pillow, I heard about it. Hiding my light under that proverbial bushel was my go-to. It made promoting my work as a teacher and writer challenging.

Friends often told me to treat myself the way I would treat my daughters or my friends. Getting ready to do something scary, like go to a writing retreat, years hence, Ellie said, "What would you tell me or Maggie?"

I tried to divide myself into two people, or characters. One is nice and supportive to the other, encouraging her on during her quests.

It wasn't easy. My default had been well established; I gave and gave to my kids without thinking about how it might impinge on my life, but I fought back. I started to consider my needs more.

One day in the early stages of my recovery, Ellie said, "Mummy, can you drive me to Harvard Square? I'm going to take the subway from there into Boston."

"No, I can't. I'm grading papers," I said and wondered how this would be received. I said yes to everybody and everything. I didn't want to upset people by telling them my opinion. I also didn't know how to fight. My mother intervened in almost every sibling disagreement and told us who was right, who was wrong. This pitted us against each other.

But when I told Ellie I couldn't drive her, she just shrugged her shoulders and said, "Okay."

Maggie and Ellie knew how to fight. I rarely intervened, only when it got physical. If I try to get involved in a fight now, they tell me to back off. I wanted them to be so much more than I was. I wanted them to be confident women, who liked themselves and knew how to ask for what they wanted and stood up for themselves.

I had never spoken up about the undercooked burgers and steaks Matt made for me. He loved rare, but I liked medium. "Matt, can you please make sure my burger is cooked through? Thanks," I said one evening. He just looked surprised but said, "Okay."

When we went to New Hampshire for a weekend, I made a point of sitting in the most comfortable chair in the house, where Matt often sat. I was used to relinquishing my spot to others. Everyone else deserved the chair or couch at home.

And I laughed. I laughed about my future with Matt after both kids were gone. There were times when I looked at him and thought, *Oh my God, really? What would we talk about?* And then, there were times when I remembered the dinners out, the movies, the dogs, and the traveling, and I realized, *Oh, this will actually be fun.*

But it was going to be work to establish myself as someone other than "just" a mother.

Years later, a new therapist suggested I find five ways to identify myself which did not include mother. That was a great exercise. In no particular order: Wife, Writer, Quilter, Teacher, Lover of Dogs.

CHAPTER SIXTEEN

With one less child at home, I turned more attention to the dogs. They entertained me and kept me busy. Three was crazy. We were lucky we had Scott. He took Spray and Ezzie out for a playdate daily. Splash was too old, slow, and cranky to go anymore. He continued to sleep on top of my feet while I wrote or edited papers.

Ellie couldn't remember our family without dogs. They were just part of her life. Maggie and Ellie grew up to be dog people, so not who I was as a kid. I had not been a dog person, but it was an identity I was happy to take on.

Ironically, now that I'd raised a litter of puppies and understood the PWD temperament more, I would think twice about selling a puppy to a family with very young children. When we got Splash, I was immersed in being a mother to young children. I took him to puppy kindergarten and walked him daily, but he remained a challenge. Perhaps it had something to do with jumping out of my moving car at forty miles per hour when he was four months old. A significant smack to his head might have changed who he was at the core; then again, maybe with more time to work with him, things would have improved.

One fall day, I walked with Ellie (who was around four years old) and Splash to pick up Maggie at the end of the school day. Splash got excited and tried to jump at and attack what he thought was a cat, but in reality, was a metal statue of a cat in a neighbor's front yard. When he hit his head on it, Ellie couldn't stop laughing.

Ellie was disappointed Spray didn't sleep with her as she had fantasized. Matt was against dogs on beds when we had Splash, who often snuck onto Maggie's bed, but Matt fell in love with Spray, as did Ellie, and the next thing I knew, Matt and I were in bed, and he called Spray.

"Spray-Spray, up. Come on, Spray. Good girl. Up." He patted the bed next to him, and Spray leapt up and snuggled down.

"What the..." I said. "Since when do we allow dogs on our bed?"

Matt just smiled as Spray cuddled against him.

Before we could trust Ezzie not to pee in the house or destroy our furniture with her teeth, she slept in a crate. Eventually, we trusted her and let her out of the crate, and she too jumped on our bed. Spray slept down by our feet, while Ezzie slept by our heads, often encircling mine and scratching it to get my attention. It wasn't always so cozy.

Spray did lie on Ellie when she knew Ellie was anxious. She could read Ellie's moods and was patient when Ellie also lay her head on Spray's tummy.

Ellie loved the dogs, though, because they listened to her and didn't criticize.

"They're cuddly, and you're never alone," she said. "They'll take care of you and protect you. They make you happy, and they're free therapy. They give hugs. They love you always."

Maggie agreed. "They're your friends no matter what. They're cute and always happy. They're fun to cuddle with."

"They love me," said Matt. "They meet me at the front door every night. No one else does that anymore." When the kids were little, they had yelled, "Daddy!" followed by, "Jump, jump!" when Matt came home from work. They'd run down the stairs and stop halfway and jump into his arms.

When we bought our house in 1991, I discovered masses of broken glass in the bushes at the far end of our urban backyard, which is the shape of a large rectangle. For years, I supposed, neighborhood teens must have used the yard as a bar.

We bought the house from an estate sale. Two sisters were born and raised there; they'd lived out their adult lives and died there too. I doubt they knew their yard was the go-to place for action.

By the time we came along, the side yard was filled with irises, and the backyard was green with grass. The crabapple tree stood proudly, one long branch reaching out over the yard, a swing dangling from a branch. In spring or summer, when the trees were in full bloom, we could almost forget we were in the city.

After a few years, the branch broke during a storm, and the swing came down. A sad day for me, but my daughters don't even remember it being there. Just like their babyhoods, they don't remember some of the key elements to our family's history, like when Maggie pulled the Christmas tree down on herself when she was two. Critical memory for me. Not for her. All she remembers are the stories we tell about it.

When the girls were small, we decided to buy a jungle gym, one to last through their childhood. For years, Maggie, Ellie and their friends swung, climbed, and slid on it. They took an old keyboard and telephone up to one of the platforms and turned the jungle gym into a rocket ship.

The jungle gym was expensive, and Matt's Aunt Cynthy (his

mom's sister) and Uncle Frank, along with my mom and Dads, helped us buy it. Matt and I were happy it was a gift from all of them.

The year before Splash joined us, we hired a landscaper to work on the yard. He laid down sod and put mulch under the swing set. I had everything I had imagined for myself. I could look out the window and see the backyard I had pictured in my mind.

Then Splash arrived and demolished the sod. He excelled at destruction.

The jungle gym lasted through Maggie's high school years, though it listed to one side. The swings didn't get much use after the girls were in third grade.

It came back to life, however, when the puppies took over the backyard. They chased each other around the swing set and through the lower platforms of the tower. Maggie and Ellie even sat on the swings again while the puppies ran underneath them.

The yard quickly morphed into a dog yard with crab grass and packed dirt, dog toys and dog poop. No matter how it looked, we were lucky to have it, even after the puppies left, because walking three dogs was challenging, but opening the back door and shooing them out there was easy.

Just as the yard changed over time, so too did my home life. In the beginning, the changes were all about adding on to my life. I went from single to married, to having babies to adding dogs. I had adapted at every step of the way. Then, just when my life couldn't be any fuller, it started to empty out. After spending twenty years growing my family, suddenly I was watching it shrink. The house full of puppies and teenagers was emptying. First, the puppies left, and then Maggie.

I wondered if I would ever get used to Maggie being gone. I

missed her terribly, but my rhythm shifted, and the house sighed each time she came home to visit and then left again.

Though they don't share my DNA like my daughters, the puppies were ingrained in me. I was invested in their futures. I had brought them up, for a few months at least, so their lives reflected at least in part on me. I cared about their happiness. I liked hearing about Charlie playing in the snow and Sparky making neighborhood friends and becoming the big sister of a human baby. I loved hearing that Zazu and Henry went to the same doggie daycare and played together.

Similarly, it tore at me when I heard that Sparky had been hit by a car, Charlie had seizures, Nauset had to have eye surgery, and Teddy got kennel cough so bad the vet hospitalized him, thinking it was something much worse. I worried alongside their new owners. Sandy was right; we were connected to them for life.

No matter how much I missed the puppies when they left our house, they were doing the appropriate thing, moving on to homes where they could get the love and attention they needed. I didn't want to keep ten dogs. Three were plenty.

The grief over their departure abated quickly, just as the grief over Maggie's initial departure lessened. I would never not long for Maggie or the little pups, but I incorporated that wanting into my life. I missed the little pups, not the grown-up dogs, and it's my family as it *was* that I missed. Living with adult children, I imagined, might be complicated. I began to pay attention to my needs— exercising more, quilting, seeing friends, but most importantly, my life was not dictated by meals and carpools. As much as I had loved those years, it was nice to have me back again.

I remembered the puppies living in our house, playing with each other and tumbling over each other, and then I'd drive by Map a couple of blocks away on Lakeview Avenue and stop to say hi.

I caught several glimpses of Map just as Maggie left for school, and the timing didn't escape my notice. Map gave me the warmest hellos a dog could give. He leaped and licked and came close to knocking me over. He was a big, powerful dog. He was handsome but looked and acted like a giant Muppet, much like his smaller sister, Ezzie.

Seeing him during the year tugged at my heart, but as spring fought to show its warm face through the rain, I stopped saying hi to him. I had to let go. His attention made me feel important and needed, but it was time for him to sever the ties with me. I started admiring him from a distance. I smiled seeing him walk proudly up the street and wondered if anyone ever stopped to comment on how stately he looked.

For the first two years after the puppies left us, we held reunions in November, when Maggie came home to see Ellie's fall play. One of these reunions was even written up in the local Cambridge paper, complete with photographs. We met in a dog park at Danehy Park, where Maggie and Ellie used to play soccer. The dog park was fenced in and consisted of sandy pebbles that absorbed urine well. It was very dusty, but it was large enough that dogs could leap and run and get some decent exercise.

When the dogs reunited, especially the first year, they gravitated to each other and played in pairs, recognizing the buddies they had played with at our house. Charlie and Nauset jumped on top of each other; Meeko and Scar ran together. Zazu pranced in like a king, and Map ran amok. Ezzie tried to stake her claim to Spray staying close to her and growling at pups who came close, but

Spray batted her with her paw a couple of times to tell her to get a grip. Everyone had returned home, briefly.

Friends and acquaintances frequently asked if we would breed again. Some of the owners wanted second dogs; some of their friends wanted first dogs. They met people who fell in love with their dogs and wanted to know where they came from.

My answer changed daily.

Genetically, Spray and Brady created great puppies. We had escaped major health issues, including dead puppies, and we had raised the puppies well during the time we had them in our house. When I see photos of the dogs with their owners, I see how happy they've made their families, and I know I did a good thing. My family helped create larger loving families. We were responsible for some happy people and dogs.

About a year after the puppies were born, we spayed Spray. She had gone through two or three more heat cycles, which she didn't need to, and had created more mess in the house, which I tried to ignore. We could have spayed her right away, but I couldn't stand the thought. It was so final. I wanted to breed her again, despite the irrationality and irony of it. I couldn't bear the thought that my family was done with this adventure, that we'd never do it again. I didn't want to make such a permanent statement by spaying her. Once she was spayed, we were done. There'd be no going back. But even as I looked back with longing, I had to look forward. I wanted more time with my family.

When I lay in bed with Maggie right after she was born, I daydreamed about how much fun the pregnancy and delivery had been, despite the fear and pain. I wanted to do it again. We had Ellie.

Then, I wanted another. I wanted a big, chaotic family. But I was sick with Epstein-Barr virus around the time we could have had a third child, and we were never sure it made sense financially or practically. We became lax about birth control and just figured whatever happened, happened. I had all the baby clothes in the basement ready to go if needed, but we didn't. They're still there if Maggie or Ellie ever want them. There was no "oops" baby for us.

It was always in Spray's best interest health-wise to get spayed, but before we could do it, she developed a cystic growth that was cottage-cheesy and worrisome around one of her teats. We tried to reduce it with hot compresses and medicine. The vet recommended that it be excised and sent to a lab for pathology testing.

Matt loved Spray so much that the thought of anything happening to her upset him, and he voted to have her spayed as soon as possible. Our roles had shifted. Suddenly, he was voting for spaying.

Spray really did need to be spayed. That was obvious.

But I stalled. I forgot to make the appointment, and she went into heat.

I rescheduled a month out, and Spray and I arrived early as required.

"Spray?"

"Yes."

"And she hasn't had anything to eat or drink since last night?"

"Oh, no," I said. How could I? I blew it once again.

I grabbed Spray by the leash, and after making yet another appointment, we left the office.

Spray went into heat one more time, and then Ezzie got kennel cough and exposed her, so we had to delay yet another appointment.

Finally, I took her in. I was sad. I wanted Matt to do this. If he hadn't been so gung ho in the beginning, we would have just spayed her at six months, and I wouldn't be feeling so ambivalent and despondent at this point. Basically, I was just confused. I had to get a grip.

I worried about her all day, calling the vet between my Emerson classes. Not surprisingly, she was fine.

When I bemoaned the sadness of it all to Matt, he reminded me that even if we could breed Spray again, it wouldn't be the same. What had made the experience so special was doing it with Maggie and Ellie. It was a family adventure. If we decided to breed again, it would be a couple's adventure. It would be with Ezzie. Spray was done.

Three years after Maggie left, Ellie packed for her own college adventure. She had visited fifteen colleges, all with theater programs. She fell in love with Emerson's, auditioned, and was accepted early. She committed to attend right away.

When Ellie and Maggie were little and they had a day off from school but I didn't, I brought them to Emerson with me. They sat in an empty classroom next to the one in which I was teaching. I provided them with paper, crayons, and coloring books to keep them busy. On one of these days, the students in my class started pointing behind me. A piece of paper slid into the classroom under the door.

"I am so sorry," I said to the class. "My kids are next door and according to this note, they're bored." The students invited Maggie and Ellie in to meet them. Everyone was in awe of each other.

Maggie said at the end of the day, "I want to go to college here."

The concept intrigued me, but I said, "You say that now, but you won't when you're ready to go." I was right.

When I said goodbye to Ellie in her stripped-down Emerson dorm room her freshman year, I wasn't overcome with desperate sadness the way I had been with my goodbye to Maggie. While she did leave the state as she wanted to, Ellie decided to go to Emerson after all.

While some moms fear the day their youngest will leave, for me, my family was permanently changed when Maggie left. Even with the three left behind, we were different. When Ellie left, I was more prepared. I didn't want to live in the past.

I prepared for the day my house would be filled with Matt, me, the dogs, and memories. Maybe breeding Ezzie would be an adventure Matt and I could undertake together. I wanted to know that life without children could be exciting again. We would take care of a new litter by ourselves. The girls wouldn't be around to help, but we'd learn to depend on each other more. Ezzie would be a different kind of mother than Spray—perhaps more energetic?

Many unknowns lurked as Matt and I prepared for a home without children. Instead of fearing those unknowns, I tried to embrace them. I was eager to see where Maggie and Ellie would end up, and I was curious to see what the next phase of my life would deliver.

To prepare for Ellie's departure to college, I started another quilt. This time, the pattern wasn't as traditional as Maggie's around-the-world one. It was more contemporary, and the colors were completely different. Ellie has always loved purple. But as she got older, she liked subtle purple. Her batik quilt had lilac, blue, green—also representative of the Vineyard.

On Ellie's move-in day, I had my shit together. After I made Ellie's bed, we covered it with the new quilt I had finished on time. I got one photo of her, hair in a messy bun standing next to her bed,

before she said, "Mummy, stop with the photos." While she wasn't
eager to say goodbye, she wanted to get on with the next act. I didn't
want to leave, either, but I would survive this time. Plus, I'd probably run into her on campus once in a while.

Ellie lived in a suite with four other students. There were two
doubles and one single, a common space, a tiny kitchen area, and
a bathroom. The best part was her view. She looked out over the
Boston Common and could see the gold dome of the State House.

"Enjoy this, Ellie," I said. "You'll never have a view like this again."

"How do you know?" Ellie asked. "That's not optimistic."

On our way back to our car after dropping Ellie off, Matt and
I passed a woman leaning against the Steinway Piano store, talking
into her cellphone and sobbing. I wanted to hug her and say, "It'll
be okay. I survived. You can too."

Ellie made it quite clear she didn't want to see or talk to us. "I want
to pretend I'm far away, like Ohio. I don't want to hear from you
or see you for six weeks," she said. Matt and I looked at each other
and raised our eyebrows. Really? This was different. We wondered
where the idea came from, but it made sense. She just wanted space.
We honored her request.

I was at Emerson twice a week teaching my writing classes, and
trying hard not to look for Ellie in the lines of students at Dunkin'
Donuts or those coming out of Starbucks across the street, though
I did wonder which one she liked more.

I didn't Facebook stalk. I didn't cry endlessly. I had started to
recreate who I was. I was writing more, spending more time with
Matt and with the dogs. I missed Ellie, but the pain wasn't nearly
as acute as it had been with Maggie. Not only was she nearby, but

I was also more prepared for the goodbye. The first one had been a doozy.

As the six weeks ended, Ellie met with us for coffee—with Matt on Tuesday mornings, after a meeting he had in the Transportation Building and before her morning classes. I visited with her on Thursday afternoons after my classes were over.

We sat in the cavernous food court in the Transportation Building as businesspeople, students, security guards, and children streamed around us while we ate donuts and drank coffee. The smell of pizza and Chinese food mingled as we chatted about how she was adapting to her new life. I learned about her roommates and friends she was making; we talked about the classes she enjoyed, like Scene Painting.

She was, however, having a harder time than she had let on. She was more homesick than I knew. She told Maggie, and while Maggie did hint at it to me, no one wanted to worry me—but later, when she was better, Ellie told me what the beginning had been like. She was probably concerned she could send me into the same hole I'd went down with Maggie.

"I miss you," she said. "I don't like being far away from you. I want to see you and the doggies."

Both girls always missed the dogs. But I learned from listening to my students, they all missed their pets. Sometimes the students said they missed their parents, but more often, it was a dog or a cat. Missing dogs wasn't as complicated as missing parents; plus, dogs can't FaceTime.

As Ellie adjusted to life away from home, I settled into a calmer house with Matt and the three dogs. The dogs still required our attention, which was a good thing.

Splash continued to age, and his incontinence grew worse. We pulled up all the rugs in the house and cleaned up after his messes. He barked with a hoarse voice, which Jay could imitate perfectly. He stood at the top of the stairs when the doorbell rang or when Matt came home from work. He no longer went down them to meet Matt at the door.

Spray did, though. While Splash stood still, Spray charged the front door, hurling herself at it whenever someone was on the other side. The plexiglass held.

Ezzie refused to grow up. Ezzie headbutted her way into any grouping where Spray was getting attention. Ezzie, albeit cute, was an attention-seeker. "Ezzie, we see you," I'd say. "Don't worry, I love you too." I reached one hand to pat Spray's head while stroking Ezzie's back with the other.

She continued to run across the living room, springing from the coffee table onto the couch next to me, Matt, or Spray. Ezzie and Spray would then bookend the sofa, lying on the back cushions. The coffee table became more scratched than my mother would have approved of, but as was true with everything in the house, it was used and loved and a marker of our family life.

I was always impressed and a little envious of those with neat, clean, organized homes—where shoes came off at the front door, and indoor shoes went on. But that wasn't me. I wanted to see the fullness that life dealt us. I wanted the family that contained a loveable mess, with my elephant collection, books, shoes, boots, and dog toys scattered around the home.

Ellie's freshman year was Maggie's senior year, and as usual, Matt and I spent much of the fall at Vassar watching field hockey games. Vassar was having the most successful season the team had had in decades, and Maggie played her personal best, winning numerous accolades and honors for her goal tending. For the first time in history, the team made it to the league playoffs and played away against their nemesis, Skidmore, in the brisk November weather. Every time Skidmore scored, the Skidmore parents rang a cowbell and screamed and hollered so loudly that even Matt with his deep voice and chants couldn't compete. Vassar lost.

After cleaning up in the locker room, the team came to the bus in the parking lot, where parents had brought food for the players to take on the ride back to school. Girls cried. The coach cried. Parents said goodbye, knowing the next time they'd see each other would be at graduation or never. The seniors were done.

Matt and I drove the four hours back to Boston in silence. Maggie's college career was coming to an end. Ellie's was just starting. Our lives were in such a place of transition, it was hard to know where we fit.

On weekends, we often watched movies. Our life as sports parents was done. Just as college athletes' lives abruptly ended when they played their last game, so too did the lives of those who watched them from the time they were tikes, running up and down a field in a clump of little beings. Once again, my identity was shifting.

Jay had moved into our two-room apartment downstairs, and we tried to balance our privacy with his. He ate dinner with us on some nights, after working in sales with a start-up software company. When he wasn't working, which seemed to be all the time, he played semi-pro football a couple of times a week. We were proud of him but also worried because we didn't want him to get hurt.

Jay was—and remains—a dog whisperer, which made having him over especially fun, because the three dogs loved him. He was patient and kind, got down on the floor to play with them gently, and he knew how to turn his back when they tried to jump on him. He never raised his voice. He had a natural ability that made them gravitate to him whenever he was in the house. Ezzie, in particular, loved him and spent hours hanging out with him on the couch or roughhousing on the floor.

When Jay didn't eat with us, Matt and I ate fried egg and bacon sandwiches, mostly on English muffins. Matt put cheese in his. On other nights, we got takeout from Full Moon or Village Kitchen. We liked the simplicity of our lives. We each had our own TV shows—I watched *NCIS*, *NCIS L.A.*, or *Grey's Anatomy*, and Matt watched *Game of Thrones*, *Blacklist*, *Orphan Black*, or *Broadchurch*. We took turns grabbing a dog or two for company. Matt watched downstairs in what had been the puppy room, and I turned my shows on in the red room. Matt had more sophisticated tastes when it came to movies and TV shows. He and Maggie loved the same shows and talked incessantly about them. I couldn't bear the suspense they loved. I needed to know everything was going to turn out okay on the shows, that the bad guys got caught.

Ellie's first year ended, and suddenly we were at Maggie's graduation. There we were—Jay, Dads, GrandBob, Tia and Casey, Matt, Ellie, and me, sitting on a hill on a hot May day, slathering on sunscreen. I was surprised by how emotional I got watching Maggie parade past us to receive her diploma. I wasn't surprised, however, by her declining mood or mine as the day wore on and she moved four years of belongings from her group house to two station wagons and Jay's Jetta.

Her tears flowed when she said goodbye to Tillan. She was moving to Texas, Maggie to Boston. When would they see each other again?

I didn't know then, however, that Maggie's return home was

going to be short-lived, and I'd have to say goodbye all over again in a few months. But I was getting better at it.

The couple at the quilt store in New Hampshire were right. My kids would boomerang back. Maggie came home more than I ever did in college. Friends with older children told me about their kids coming home after graduating from college, because they couldn't afford their own places. I shouldn't get so sad, they said.

Even if Maggie and Ellie returned home for financial reasons, it would be temporary. They were moving forward.

I didn't want them to mimic our neighbors, whose three children were homeschooled and never left the nest—ever. In their forties, they lived with their parents and helped them run their businesses— a boarding house, a card company, and parade performances.

As much as I missed my children, I was also proud of them and their accomplishments. It was fun to watch Maggie shine in field hockey and to start a career in the entertainment industry. I was excited watching Ellie embrace her college experience with such enthusiasm.

Nothing was over. My life was just changing shape.

I cried the day our jungle gym came down, thanks to contractors who took it apart while they were shingling our house. But once the shock wore off, when I looked out in the backyard, I didn't notice the absence of the jungle gym. I saw a playground for dogs.

Maggie moved home after graduation and flitted between her room in our house and Jay's apartment downstairs, eventually set- tling into the tiny rental of two rooms. We didn't make it to the Vineyard much that summer because everyone—including Ellie, who was involved with Boston Children's Theater—had work at home. Maggie was at Full Moon and working as a production assistant on the film *Black Mass*. Jay continued his work in sales at the start-up software company. While I missed the Vineyard, tennis, my friends, and Dads, I didn't want to miss the rare opportunity to be with the girls, Jay, and Matt. I took pottery lessons in town and started taking Ezzie for the same genetic tests that Spray had done, as we were gearing up to have a new litter for FayerWaves.

In the end of August, Splash died. Ellie and her then-boyfriend came home one day, and when they opened the back door for Splash to come in, he collapsed and couldn't stand up and get inside. They pulled him into the back room where the puppies had been born, and he stayed there. I knew Splash was going to die someday. When he was particularly annoying, I even recommended, "Go to the light, Splash. It's okay."

He didn't take my hints and became more and more infirmed. He was fifteen and a half years old, after all, but I couldn't believe we had actually gotten to the point where we were going to say goodbye; goodbye to the pain in the butt who had been our best friend.

I went to TJ Maxx and bought him a dog bed, so he had something to lie on besides the cold, hard floor. We called the vet and made an appointment for the next day. Splash barely made it onto the bed, lying half on it and half on the floor. He couldn't be moved.

Dr. Binder—who had replaced Dr. Emara and was equally as kind and compassionate—and her assistant, Brad, came to our house, and we circled around Splash on his new striped bed with the door to the sunny, warm backyard open. We took turns telling Splash how much we loved him and thanked him for being our friend. I gave each person space to talk to him without listening in too intently.

"Splash," I whispered into his ear. "Thanks for being there when Gabby (my mom) was dying. Thanks for being there for Maggie when she needed a friend." I walked out onto the back porch and cried in the warm air. My children were grown up. Goodbye to my years of being a hands-on mom. Splash's reign was over.

Matt cut a piece of Splash's hair for us to keep in a plastic bag. We laid our hands on Splash's thinning hair and pet him, tears streaming down our faces.

"Are you ready?" Dr. Binder asked.

Heads nodded. No words.

"This shot will put him to sleep," she said as she injected it.

More tears flowed.

"This shot will stop his heart."

I wanted him to leap up and annoy us. He had given me such a headache, and yet he had followed me wherever I went in the house, laid his body on my feet as I worked at my computer, and loved me.

We had shut Spray and Ezzie in Matt's office down the hall, per Dr. Binder's instruction, while we took care of Splashy, but when he was gone, Dr. Binder said to bring them out.

"Let them smell their friend so they know he is gone, and they won't look for him," Dr. Binder said.

Maggie and Ellie brought them out on leashes. They walked around Splash a couple of times, sniffed him, and sauntered away. They never looked for him again.

We wrapped Splash's body in a towel, and Matt carried it to the vet's car on the street. He whispered to Splash, "Let's go on one more walk."

We were down to two dogs and a quieter house.

CHAPTER SEVENTEEN

I didn't want to breed Ezzie while Splash was with us—it was too much for me to handle. Plus, Ezzie might calm down a little if she were a little older. Her energy was impressive.

But now that Splash was gone, we were ready to breed Ezzie. She was four years old, which was getting up there for breeding, but the new vet I saw, Dr. Kind, said if I hurried, Ezzie would do fine. Her litter might be small; the older the bitch, the smaller the litter. That was also okay. I didn't need ten puppies again.

According to the vet, Ezzie had a great temperament, which our family naturally agreed with. She was calmer, sweet, and funny. I was excited. This would be my next phase. I could get on board with this. Maggie and Jay were home to help, and Ellie was across the river at Emerson for her sophomore year. It was perfect. I couldn't have asked for more.

I came home from teaching on a Thursday afternoon in October, and Ezzie didn't run to the front door demanding attention by leaping at me while I yelled, "Get a toy!" She lay by the back French doors with a cone around her head and neck, to keep her from licking a wound on her rump. But that wasn't what stopped me.

Her brown curly mop of a head lay in vomit. Her tail thumped on the floor when she saw me, but she barely moved. She eventually roused herself, I cleaned her, and we went upstairs where she regained some enthusiasm. By the end of the evening, however, after Matt came home, she had thrown up a couple more times and didn't look too perky.

"I think I should take her to Angell," Matt said as we sat in the living room after dinner. Angell Memorial, an animal hospital in Jamaica Plain, was at least twenty minutes away.

"She'll be okay," I said. "It's probably some stomach thing. I'll take her to Cushing in the morning if she's not better."

Morning came, and she wasn't better. I took her to Dr. Binder in Belmont.

Ezzie liked to sit on the chairs in the waiting area for her appointments. She sat bolt upright waiting her turn, just like her mother sat in the armchair in our living room. This day, she wasn't as enthused.

After Ezzie and I were in one of the examining rooms, Dr. Binder opened Ezzie's mouth to look at her gums and then palpated her stomach.

"I need to do X-rays and blood work, okay?" She asked.

"Sure," I said, a bit concerned. Dr. Binder was direct. She wasn't chatting with me as she usually did, asking about my family.

When the results were back, Dr. Binder explained that Ezzie's spleen and liver were enlarged. A lot. Her white cell count was elevated, and her gums were white, meaning she was losing blood. None of this was good news. She needed to go to the hospital.

"Most likely, she has a tick-borne disease or leptospirosis," said Dr. Binder, who explained that leptospirosis was a bacterial infection often picked up by dogs when they roll around in or sniff urine left by infected animals. There was a slight chance, she said, Ezzie could have cancer. But most likely, a heavy dose of antibiotics would take care of whatever she had. It might mean no puppies, however, which made me sadder than I expected. I was tired of losing control of my life.

I called Matt and relayed Dr. Binder's concerns.

"I'll see you at Angell," he said.

Matt met me at the huge antiseptic animal hospital, with which we were familiar. Our dogs had been there many times after ingesting grapes, chocolate, aspirin, and numerous other things they weren't supposed to eat. Splash had spent a week there years earlier when he had vestibular disease. He was so dizzy, he walked like a drunk man, and we couldn't take care of him at home. The Angell staff was smart and compassionate.

We were ushered into an examining room with Ezzie. The vet repeated what Dr. Binder had said. She took Ezzie's leash and led her out for more testing, assuring us it was most likely leptospirosis.

When she returned, she had bad news. Ezzie did have cancer. But with chemo, she could live for a couple of years. We had pet insurance. We could do this. No puppies, but we had bouncy Ezzie. We could figure this out. She would have to stay over for a while to get her blood levels up, start on chemo, and then she'd be good to go.

That didn't happen.

After even more testing, the vet told us Ezzie's cancer was multicentric lymphoma, and she actually only had a few months. I wanted to take her home.

"Let's take her to the Vineyard," I suggested to Matt. "Let her walk on the beach even if it's too cold for the water." I wanted her to sleep on top of my head in bed, her favorite position. I wouldn't even mind her scratching my scalp. I wanted to watch TV with her. She wasn't even five years old. She was supposed to be a mom, not dead.

I didn't have time to adjust. One minute Ezzie was leaping off our coffee table, and the next she could barely sit up. We were waiting for her genetic test results but had no reason for fear. There had been no symptoms, no warning signs. She bounced around the house and then boom, she didn't. I called Dr. Kind later to say we weren't following through with the breeding, which broke my heart. The vet was kind and gentle on the phone.

"I'm so sorry. This is something I've seen before. It's sad," she said.

Not only had we spent money, time, and energy on getting Ezzie ready for breeding, but also, after weeks of searching, I had finally, maybe, found a stud dog for her. When I got the email back from the other breeder that yes, she was interested in talking with me further about making a match between Ezzie and her dog, I was thrilled. We were moving forward. This plan was going to fill my days and keep me busy when my house emptied out. Instead of being sad about everyone leaving, I had looked forward, with a little trepidation, to Ezzie and puppies, with Matt. Now that plan was gone.

I wanted Ezzie to be okay. We wanted to love her as much as possible during her last months.

We left her at Angell, where they started her on a chemo drip. When we returned that evening for visiting hours, we found her in an oxygen crate. Her breathing was labored. We took turns sitting in the crate with her, bent over in contorted positions. She wasn't particularly perky, but she thumped her tail on the ground a bit when we came in.

Matt, Maggie, and I visited her twice a day. Ellie came when she could leave school. For three days, her condition improved with chemo, steroids, and a blood transfusion. On Monday morning, she had improved enough that the medical team moved her into an

open run. She was digging at her bed when we arrived. She was energetic Ezzie, and her tail swished back and forth when she saw us.
Jay, who loved Ezzie and her spunkiness, came with us Monday
evening. We were excited to see Ezzie, who we thought would be
home soon. But we were wrong. Ezzie was worse. She had started
bleeding internally and could barely lift her tail to say hi. If I had to
guess how she felt, it was sad and scared. She curled up and barely
came to say hi.

"If she's going to die, I want to bring her home," I said to the
vet on call. Ezzie needed to be with her family, and we needed to
be with her. I didn't want her to be alone in a cold concrete room.
Late at night, we got the call. We should come and get her. Around
one a.m. Tuesday morning, Maggie and I drove back to Angell and
picked up Ezzie. It was clear to the vets at Angell that Ezzie wasn't
going to make it. The transfusions weren't working.

When we got her home, she ran into the house, jumped on
every couch and bed, her brown curls bouncing, and lay in all her
favorite spots. She was dying. We wanted to spend a day with
her and made an appointment with our vet to revisit our house
Wednesday afternoon, about six weeks from when she had been
there for Splash. We planned to say goodbye to Ezzie after we had
a chance to drench her in our love.

Matt went to work at the airport Tuesday morning, dragging
his feet. He didn't want to leave but thought he'd have Wednesday
to spend at home with Ezzie. I canceled my classes. By that afternoon, after Matt came home early, Ezzie was bleeding rectally.

After a call to Dr. Binder—with whom we had stayed in touch
while Ezzie was at Angell—she told us it was probably time to say
goodbye.

Ezzie was going to suffer if we didn't. We couldn't wait until

Wednesday. Ellie made her way home from Emerson. We owed it to Ezzie to help her. If we didn't euthanize her, her spleen could explode, which would be painful, explained Dr. Binder. But apart from the bleeding, which was substantial, she didn't seem to be in pain and wandered to each of us, giving us all a moment to be with her. She even had a chance to say goodbye to Scott when he brought Spray home from a playdate.

Ezzie went to the top of the stairs and looked down at Scott, who climbed partway up and leaned in to say goodbye. Scott will tell you, the worst part of his job as dog-walker is saying a last goodbye to the dogs he spends his days with.

He had seen Ezzie as a newborn pup and watched her grow up, taking her for daily playdates. Leaning on the staircase, he pet her and said, "Bye, Ezzie. You have been fun. I'll miss you."

We took her to Cushing Square Vet in Belmont, where we gathered around her on a blanket in the warm fall sun. Spray, Jay, Matt, Maggie, Ellie, and I surrounded her, but she didn't move onto the blanket and lie down, so Jay walked around to the other side and called her.

"Are you her favorite?" asked Dr. Binder.

Everyone was Ezzie's favorite. That's what made Ezzie so special. She loved each one of us like we were the only one in the room, but she sure did love Jay, who played with her every chance he got.

Ezzie wagged her tail, walked towards Jay, and lay down. All our hands rested on her and our tears bathed her. Dr. Binder only had to give her one shot. She was that sick. She died fast.

Again, Matt carried a wrapped body, this time into the vet's office. We drove home in two cars, in silence, and arrived to a house filled with Ezzie reminders. Over the next couple of days, I picked up her toys. I threw some away and boxed up the others for the basement, although I'm not sure why. In six weeks, we had gone from a crazy house of three dogs to a lonely house of one.

That night and for many more to come, I slept with a blanket that smelled of Ezzie. I missed Ezzie on my head.

After Ezzie died, Maggie and Jay went to Los Angeles for a Vassar alumni panel on the TV and film industry so Maggie, who had double majored in film and psychology, could hear about the world out there.

They returned a week later to tell Matt and me they were moving in January. "What?" I must have asked. "Really?" I knew moving was a possibility, but I thought I had at least a year with them at home. But, Maggie had already made a contact for a possible internship out there, and Jay could keep his current job as a salesperson with a software company because he worked remotely.

"How exciting," I told them in our kitchen, as I forced a smile. "I am so proud of you." I was. This would be a great adventure for them. It was also a good way for them to establish themselves as a unit, away from family intrusions, like me.

Matt was equally effusive about the move, but I knew he was going to miss his buddies just as much as me. There went any chance of Maggie and Jay going to football games with him. I thought I might throw up. That was it, they were gone. My card games of Pounce, and Spite & Malice, were over.

Friends tried to make me feel better by telling me Maggie and Jay wouldn't stay out there forever, but even if they moved back at some point, they would never live in our apartment again. The phase with them home for the breeding was being replaced with a phase of me being on my own, more independent. I could do this, I said to myself, while holding back the tears.

A couple of weeks later, I went back to our vet to pick up Ezzie's ashes. I walked through the waiting room area, where owners and dogs sat for their appointments. There was even a puppy I couldn't help but pet. I walked up to Evan, the receptionist, one of the kindest people. "I'm here for Ezzie," I choked out.

He looked so sad when he handed me the bag with the box with Ezzie's ashes. Two boxes of ashes now sat on our bookcase. One had a photo of baby Splash and Maggie on the beach; the other had a close-up of Ezzie's face. We had planned on burying them under trees on the Vineyard, but years later, they remain in our TV room keeping us company.

I missed Ezzie. Watching Maggie and Jay clean out their tiny apartment and Maggie's bedroom in our house and box and bag their clothes and kitchen appliances didn't help me feel better.

They added to our overflowing basement with cartons of winter clothes and household items they couldn't fit in their car or didn't need in L.A. Their stuff in the basement was comingled with years of Playmobil, plastic figurines, our collection of holiday books, and, of course, baby clothes.

Maggie and Jay chatted about their upcoming move excitedly. They were going to move in with family in Santa Monica, and Maggie would start her internship. Jay started a successful dog-walking business, and four years later, they rescued their own dog, Brody, a spaniel-mix. He was doted on by Maggie and Jay, and together they turned a scared dog with a history of abuse and neglect into a loving member of their family.

They were moving into their future. But they didn't like the packing part or the saying goodbye part.

I definitely was not a fan of the goodbye, but this one would be different. I wasn't going to fall into the hole again. I was done with being depressed. So when I felt myself slipping, I thought about what would make me happy, what would fill that void.

I needed a puppy.

Within a week, I started calling breeders for a new Portuguese water dog puppy. Who knew, fifteen years earlier when we got Splash, I would turn into such a dog person? It wasn't just that I wanted a dog; I missed the nurturing I had done for so long. A puppy would need my love and attention, with the girls gone. They would only need a long-distance mom.

A puppy couldn't replace Ezzie or Maggie and Jay, but it sure could help fill the void that was growing in my heart. But no one would give me one. When breeders discovered we had bred Spray without putting her through dog shows, they were horrified. Spray wasn't a champion. Even though she was the product of champions, she hadn't gone through the qualifications to make herself one.

"She's my champion," Matt said.

Some breeders were concerned we might want to breed again. The thought had crossed our minds, as Matt and I didn't really know what we were going to do next. Ellie was ensconced at Emerson, and Maggie and Jay were leaving soon. Breeding could replace the loneliness. I called every breeder I could find while I watched Maggie and Jay pack and plan for a month.

Finally, my luck changed.

I finally found a breeder who would work with me on the south shore. I just wanted a pet. I didn't need to breed again. I just wanted to hold a puppy in my lap.

She was having a litter and surprised me, as she wondered if

I wanted to share a puppy. The puppy would live with us, but she would borrow her to show and then to breed.

Yes, Matt and I said. This would give us something to do as a couple. We could learn a new world, like the Nightingales had done in their later years. We would go to the dog shows, we would get the puppy involved in water sports—diving and swimming. We could be crazy dog people.

In another month—a few weeks before Maggie and Jay moved—the breeder's dog, gave birth to her litter. She let us come when the puppies were three weeks old so Maggie and Jay could meet the pup before they moved. This was unusual and very kind.

We needed to name the pup. After a lot of back and forth we settled on Mayzie, spelled in a way to acknowledge Ezzie. No one knows how to spell it, and now years later, who really cares?

While Mayzie grew bigger and stronger at the breeder's, Maggie and Jay jammed his Jetta so full of bags and boxes there was hardly room for the two of them. On an exceptionally cold January morning, the five of us stood outside our house and hugged each other goodbye. "I love you, tons and tons," I told Maggie repeatedly.

Maggie wore her sleeping bag of a maroon down coat that hung down to her ankles, which she would need on the drive across the country but would shed once she reached L.A. Despite the cold winter weather, they planned their trip through Niagara Falls to Chicago, and Madison to Salt Lake City, partly to see family and partly because it was hopefully friendlier than the south might be to an interracial couple. I worried about their safety, especially Jay's because he could be stopped by a cop and killed.

Before they left, we took out our phones and my good camera and started to memorialize this momentous occasion. We shared a desperate need for everyone to have a picture with the movers, just like we had done when the puppies left our home. I can now scroll through photos of Jay and Ellie; Jay, Maggie and Ellie, with Matt photo-bombing behind them. There was one of Maggie and Jay standing by Jay's Jetta, and one of me and Mags, and of course one of Maggie and Matt.

Ellie cried more than I did, if that was possible. The continuity she'd had with Maggie was gone. For years, Ellie and Maggie were each other's go-to person, and that was changing. This was harder on Ellie than I had anticipated.

Knowing how important this move was for Maggie and Jay, made it slightly easier to wave goodbye as they drove up the street and honked their horn as they turned onto Huron Ave.

Unlike when she was at Vassar, there were no school vacations to look forward to this time. This departure had no end in sight. I was so tired of goodbyes. As much as I wanted them to stay squished in the apartment downstairs, work in the neighborhood, and play cards with me, they needed to grow as a couple, and as individuals, and they needed to get away from family to start their own lives.

I followed their trip through their Instagram posts as they went north through the freezing cold. Maggie posted photos of them at Niagara Falls, where she wore a Patriots hat and Jay had on a Dallas Cowboys one. In another photo, they smiled from Chicago. In Madison, Wisconsin, Maggie skated on a pond on a frigid day while she and Jay stayed with Matt's sister, Jane, and her husband, Joe.

I checked in with Maggie regularly to make sure all was good. It always was, except at Omaha's Henry Doorly Zoo, where a white man stared Jay down across one of the indoor animal pens. Maggie and Jay felt unwelcome and uncomfortable.

I liked being part of their journey, seeing who they visited and what they were seeing. I wasn't stalking anyone this time. The posts were intended for everyone to see, through which to live vicariously.

When they reached L.A. and the energy of their trip ended, I was deflated. They had arrived at their permanent destination. I sat around feeling sorry for myself for the next month, missing Maggie and Jay, listening to the quiet from downstairs. The loneliness burned.

After Maggie and Jay moved out, Scott moved into the small apartment and has remained our dogs' best friend.

Matt spent most of his time in front of the TV, where he could escape his feelings of loss. He watched football and his favorite scary TV shows, which he and Maggie used to watch together. Maybe this was his way of staying connected to her.

"Maybe I should sell the tickets," he suggested. He wasn't sure keeping the Patriots tickets made sense anymore.

"No, you'll regret it," I replied. "Ellie is still here, and Maggie may move back. Sell individual games, but keep the season tickets."

On February 1, Matt visited Maggie and Jay in L.A. for Super Bowl XLIV to watch the game. In Boston, we were about to get hit with the second string of blizzards that buried Boston in up to seven feet of snow that year.

While they were getting ready for kickoff, I drove to the south shore with Spray in the passenger seat, to get Mayzie. The front yard was solid ice, very slippery. I was eager and scared about bringing this tiny puppy home alone. You'd have thought I'd never had a puppy in my house before, not the three I'd raised to adult dogs or the ten I'd helped whelp and taken care of until they moved to their forever homes.

I introduced Mayzie to Spray out in the cold, letting Spray smell Mayzie in the breeder's arms.

After they sniffed each other and I figured they would be okay, I put Mayzie in a crate in the back of the station wagon. I turned the radio on so I couldn't hear her cry.

Once home, I carried Mayzie—a tiny black PWD with a white chest and one white sock—upstairs to our red TV room, where I plopped her on the couch with me. I put a Patriots hat on her, and together with Spray, we watched the Patriots beat the Seahawks.

EPILOGUE

Mayzie brought joy back into my life. I call her my "happy dog." I taught Mayzie fetch by throwing a toy down the hallway, and as a little pup, she scampered down the hall, got it and brought it back. It was too cold and snowy outside.

Mayzie also turned out to be one of the coziest dogs. She will lie on the back of a couch, on a cushion like Spray and many PWDs do, but then crawl into a lap—mostly Matt's. She is sweet and funny, turning in circles the way Spray did or ripping apart an empty yogurt container.

She is the best tail-wagger I've ever met. She wags it vigorously. It thumps the ground as she waves it back and forth to tell you that she loves you or wants to play a game. Sometimes she wags it in a circle. Like Ezzie, she too likes to sleep on top of my head in bed, but she doesn't scratch me as much.

In the years since Mayzie has joined our family, change keeps happening. I know now there is no such a thing as a static family. Nor should there be.

As Maggie and Jay shed their winter clothes, and Maggie started her internship, we tried to housetrain Mayzie, who we could only really take out in the backyard, because the sidewalks were too narrow to walk down from the high snow drifts on either side.

Matt dug a circle in the five feet of snow so Mayzie and Spray could run in it—the snow would bury Mayzie, and even Spray had trouble carving a path in it. Mayzie learned to pee and poop in that circle, and when we did take her on walks around the neighborhood after the snow had melted a bit, Mayzie sniffed and scurried around front yards, but she waited until we returned home and ran in the backyard to do what needed to be done.

I spent more time with Ellie, visiting her while she worked at the front desk checking student IDs in one of the Emerson dorms. I brought homemade brownies and cookies to her and the security guard. Ellie had stopped hiding from me on campus.

One April day, as she was entering her dorm, the student checking her ID said, "Oh my god. You're Morgan Baker's daughter!" Ellie and I do resemble each other, and that year we both had white winter coats. I didn't advertise who my daughter was (we have different last names) but when the connection was made, I beamed. Ellie was equally happy. "Yeah, that's my mom," she remembers thinking.

On May 1, I walked into my classroom in the Walker Building before the students had arrived, to discover a bunch of flowers and a box of donuts from Blackbird Donuts at my seat. Ellie had dropped them off for my birthday.

When Maggie moved to California after graduation, she called me on her way to work almost daily. I knew then, that even if I was busy, being on the phone with her was important. During the Vassar calls, I listened to what her new life was like. During the L.A. calls, I figured out ways to keep productive—pinning a quilt, washing dishes, straightening the house. I didn't listen to those who recommended I tell her I was busy. I wanted to be there for Maggie no matter what. If I lost an hour of work time, so be it. She was more important.

Maggie started her internship at a company that produced un-scripted (reality) TV shows. She was lucky she had family there who housed her. Unpaid internships do not level the playing field for those who don't have resources to help them through the internships, and they should be banned. Maggie's internship eventually turned into a paid receptionist job. From there, she got into the Page Program at NBC/Universal, and when that ended, she landed an assistant's position in the film division of the company. Jay worked sales for several start-up software companies, started his dog walking business, and eventually became regional manager of several Stretch Lab locations. Maggie left Universal after a promotion there and now works for an established film production company.

They are both excited about their careers. Jay loves the weather and fresh produce in L.A. and is outside as much as possible, swimming, playing basketball, and riding his bike. Maggie likes it too, but she misses the East Coast and the changing seasons. In the midst of all the changing careers, they came back to the Vineyard in 2017 to get married in the field next to where Matt and I had married twenty-nine years earlier.

Ellie and Mayzie bonded because Ellie visited home a lot while at Emerson. Ellie graduated, and as a faculty member, I got to read her name at the huge ceremony inside BU's Agganis Arena, a very different experience than Maggie's outside in the sun. Drummers brought the graduating class in, and they took their seats on the floor. Matt, Ellie, Dads, GrandBob, and Betsy sat high in the seats. When the commencement speaker finished talking, I snuck down to the waiting area, and was then escorted to the back of the stage. I stepped up to the mic at the podium just before Ellie approached. I was so proud to be part of that moment with her.

I visited Maggie and Jay a lot in the early years after they moved, but as time moved on, and after they got married, our trips slowed down.

Ellie moved into a family-owned condo in Cambridge for her senior year of college and stayed for four more years. She acted in plays on the Vineyard and in Boston. To pay the bills, she worked retail at a variety of shops.

The trouble with the future is, no one knows what it will bring. Maggie and Ellie are young and must adjust to the unknown ahead. Change sometimes comes when you don't plan for it.

When I turned sixty, an old friend reached out to see if I was interested in being part of a start-up web magazine geared to an older audience. I loved the idea of a new adventure. I became managing editor of *The Bucket*. I wrote and edited, met a lot of writers, and got to help with the mission of the magazine—to live a more fulfilling life by acknowledging and embracing your mortality. Not to stop living.

One of the most surprising shifts in our life was that Matt and I moved to Hawaii for a year for a new job for him. This was a real *Bucket*-y move. Afraid of change, as I was, I wasn't on board for this initially, but it was the right move for Matt. It turned out to be one of the best adventures we've been on. Choosing to move, making a change, is different than when change was thrust upon me as a kid. Having agency in a decision made a huge difference about how I perceived the change.

All the puppies from Spray's litter are gone. Each death hit hard, harder than I anticipated. We were responsible for bringing these dogs into the world. We hadn't planned on the grieving part. The loss was not just about each puppy but also about the adventure. It is receding into our family history. But as painful as grief is, it is the cost of love. If you love hard, you'll grieve hard.

Spray, too, is no longer with us, which was a shocker. When the family gathered in L.A. for Thanksgiving 2018, Spray and Mayzie stayed with Scott in Cambridge. Scott called as we were getting ready to leave Maggie's apartment for a shopping expedition, and he said, "Spray has been lethargic all day. I'm thinking I should take her to the hospital."

"What? Why don't you wait a bit?" Then, after talking to Matt, I called back. "Take her now." Scott was already in his car with her.

The four of us got in Maggie's car to meet Tia for some shopping. We never made it. When the phone rang, we pulled over. "It doesn't look good, Morgan," Scott said.

"What do you mean?"

"They're doing compressions."

"What?"

A new voice got on the phone and introduced himself as the vet. "Her heart has stopped, and she's stopped breathing. Do you want us to continue compressions?"

"No."

Ellie leaped from the car and started screaming, scaring a UPS delivery person on the sidewalk. Tears pooled at Matt's chin, and Maggie and I stared ahead at the road in front of us.

Scott asked what we wanted him to do. Eventually, he went into the room, where they had placed Spray on a table with a blanket on her, and he put the phone to her head and we took turns saying goodbye.

Mayzie didn't have the chance to smell her the way Ezzie and Spray had said goodbye to Splash, and she continued to look for her for a long time.

The pandemic hit shortly after Matt and I had returned from Hawaii. That was an unplanned transition for the whole world. No one had any agency in that one. Ellie moved home, as her then-boyfriend went on a business trip and decided to visit his family in California and never came back. We watched a lot of TV, as did the rest of the country. *Schitt's Creek*, *Hacks*, *The Gambit*, and *All Creatures Great and Small* were some of our favorites. We played backgammon and cards.

Matt and I started walking around Cambridge; we circled Fresh Pond and walked by the Charles River on weekends. We worked out on Zoom with my trainer from our old gym that closed when the pandemic arrived. I got to see Betsy a lot on Zoom and other friends I had made from the gym.

My work with *The Bucket* slowed way down. It was difficult to embrace *The Bucket*'s mission when there was so much death in the world.

I didn't get to see my father in England or Maggie and Jay for more than a year. We lived on FaceTime, which was better than nothing. We finally saw Maggie when she surprised Ellie for her twenty-sixth birthday in March. In June, the five of us went to the Vineyard for a short week of eating, swimming, walking, and watching our newest puppy, Lily. Lily was a Christmas present for Matt and Ellie. She and Mayzie romped in the field and ran up and down the beach, and they took to the water like any good PWD.

My life as a mother has been about learning the balance between holding on and letting go. My children have always come first. I've had to pry my hands open to let them go when I really want to keep them close. I have even encouraged them to let go of me and move if necessary. I want what's best for my children to grow, even if it means I'm left behind, seemingly diminished.

I am learning that I am more than a mother. I am a quilter, writer, teacher, wife, and lover of dogs.

Bringing yet another puppy home during the pandemic, as did many other people, provided constant entertainment. Lily, we discovered, was a funny dog. She fell in love with Mayzie and liked to bolt around the living and dining rooms and back again. Mayzie sometimes chased her; other times she sat and watched.

As I observe my children moving forward in their lives, I hold onto Mayzie as she lies on top of me while we watch TV or sleeps next to me in bed.

When I think of the change that is out there, my stomach knots up, my skin gets itchy, I become short of breath and want to stay in bed with the dogs.

But encouraging my children to go for their dreams is the mature thing to do. And, as we say in my family, it's time to put on my big girl pants. It was also time for me to go after my dreams.

Those pants fit me well these days. Instead of watching my daughters on the sidelines, I've put myself on the field. I work out, write, and sew quilts. Instead of being sad that I only had a few days with my family on the Vineyard, I stayed on alone after they left and enjoyed my own companionship.

I will always be a mother, but having it be the central role in my life—with everything else tethered to it and by which I am defined—is gone. I don't wake up and worry about carpools and lunch bags. I don't worry about homework, field hockey practice, and play rehearsals. And, I do not miss that. I do miss sitting around the dining room table listening and laughing.

I'm stronger and in better shape since before kids. I'm still in therapy and on medication. I dream of not needing them, but reality reminds me that I need support, and that's okay.

I'm better at paying attention to what I need. I like time alone with my projects, and the time Matt and I share together—walking, watching TV, laughing, and playing with the dogs.

As I crossed off quilt after quilt during the pandemic, I said to Matt, "What am I going to do? I only have two more quilts to make."

"There will always be a quilt for you to make, Morg," he replied.

And, there will also always be changes.

ACKNOWLEDGEMENTS

I wrote this story for me. It was the story I was looking for when my daughters were moving out of our home and into their own lives. I wanted to make sense of that transition. And, I did. I discovered there is life after children, and it's pretty great.

This book would not have been possible without all the readers, writers, friends, family, and editors who supported and encouraged me along the way. I'm terrified of forgetting someone, but I'm human, so I probably have. If you're that person, please forgive me and know I am grateful for your help.

I owe a special debt of gratitude to Shannon Ishizaki, owner and publisher of Ten16 Press, who saw the opportunity to elevate this message of empowerment. She recognized the significance of women finding their identities in a world where it's easy to lose them to our children. Thank you to Pam Parker for your close reading, editing, and understanding, and to Kaeley Dunteman for getting the story on the cover, and thank you to Jenna Zerbel for her copyediting and keeping me organized. To the rest of the Ten16 crew, thank you for devoting your talents to this book.

This story has had many iterations and titles. I am grateful to Marcie Hershman and Sally Ryder Brady, who read very early manuscripts. Thank you to David Emblidge and his Book Publishing class at Emerson for including my book as part of the editing curriculum. To Annie Tucker, thank you for excising pieces of the story to reveal the most potent story possible. Many thanks to the Grit Sisters, Lisa and Laura Birk, for keeping me accountable during the second draft. Thank you, Sheila Bender, and all the writers I've met through your classes. Your questions always encourage me to write a richer story.

Thank you, Rebecca Steinitz, line-editor extraordinaire. Your encouragement and enthusiasm never flagged through the years. You have stood by this project since the beginning. I so appreciate your counsel.

Allison K. Williams, thank you for telling me to go deeper in the hard parts. Thank you, Dinty Moore, for showing me how to follow that "river."

Big thank yous to Trina, Betsy, Tia, Debbie, Delia, Dawn, Myriam, Tammy, Amy, and Catriona for reading drafts and cheering me on along the way. Thank you to my therapists, book group, and Emerson friends for your support during this journey.

And, to all the writer-friends I've met in person and online, I am so grateful for our connections and friendship. I am more confident and powerful as a result of this writing community. Thank you to all my co-writing buddies in the mornings and afternoons. Writing side by side with you is a joy.

Allison Lane and the Buzzworthy Lab Group, thank you for your patience and encouragement. I am not a self-promoter, but Allison worked her magic, insisted I could do it, and helped me put myself and my work out there.

A huge thank you to all my students for the past three decades. Working with you has been a thrill. You motivate and inspire me, and you make me laugh. I learn more from you than you probably realize. And, my writing has continued to evolve because of you.

Sadly, Jim and Sandy Nightingale, Spray's breeders, are no

longer with us, but their kindness, support, dog enthusiasm, and belief in our family helped us have the most fun and exciting adventure.

Thank you Splash, Spray, Ezzie, Mayzie, and Lily. You keep me laughing. You made me a dog person. Thank you for teaching me to be in the moment and open to new adventures.

Finally, and most importantly, thank you to my family—Matt, Maggie, Ellie, and Jay. Your support and encouragement buoyed me. Thank you for letting me share your stories as they intersected with mine. You are resilient, kind, smart, and very funny. Watching you navigate your own challenges is inspirational. I am who I am today because of you. You have enriched my life in ways I couldn't have predicted thirty-five years ago, when I said, "I will." I love you all.

And to you, Matt Brelis, you have always been there. Thank you for being my first and most honest reader. Thank you for believing in the book and for always believing in me, especially when I didn't. You always have my back, know how to read my mind, and no one makes me laugh like you do. I am lucky. Thank you for being my best friend.

CPSIA information can be obtained
at www.ICGtesting.com
Printed in the USA
JSHW010912130423
40240JS00005B/24